**rch into
practice**

D0279445

Research into practice

A reader for nurses and the caring professions

Edited by
Pamela Abbott and Roger Sapsford

Open University Press
Buckingham · Philadelphia

Open University Press
Celtic Court
22 Ballmoor
Buckingham
MK18 1XW

and

1900 Frost Road, Suite 101
Bristol, PA 19007, USA

First Published 1992

A catalogue record of this book is available from the British Library

Library of Congress Cataloging-in-Publication Data

Nursing research into practice : a reader for nurses and the caring
  professions / [edited Pamela Abbott and Roger Sapsford.
     p.   cm.
  Includes bibliographical references and indexes.
  ISBN 0–335–09742–1 (pbk.) — ISBN 0–335–09743–X (hbk.)
  1. Nursing—Research. I. Abbott, Pamela. II. Sapsford, Roger.
  [DNLM: 1. Nursing Research. 2. Research Design. WY 20.5 N97444]
RT81.5.N8744 1992
610.73'072—dc20
DNLM/DLC
for Library of Congress   91–46282
                                                               CIP

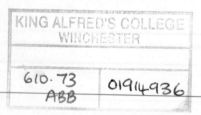
Typeset by Colset Private Limited, Singapore
Printed in Great Britain by Biddles Limited, Guildford and Kings Lynn

Contents

Preface and acknowledgements

This book is a collection of examples of research, all concerned in some way with nursing or the study of health and community care. It was compiled to accompany a textbook on research methods, *Research Methods for Nurses and the Caring Professions*, by Roger Sapsford and Pamela Abbott, but it will also stand by itself as an introduction to research. It illustrates the kind of research that can be done by a small research team or a single researcher – not 'grand projects', but small-scale investigations of theoretical issues or aspects of practice. All the chapters describe research which was done or could be done by a single researcher, without large-scale research grants (the most expensive being the statistical analysis described in Chapter 10, which requires the services of a mainframe computer). There is a great diversity of approaches: differing emphasis on description or explanation, different degrees of structures in the design, differing appeals to the authority of science or the authenticity of empathic exploration. The chapters also show the limitations typical of small-scale projects carried out with limited resources; though each is good of its kind, each also reflects the experience of applied research as it occurs in practice, as opposed to how it tends to look when discussed in methods textbooks.

Six of the chapters have appeared in previous edited collections, and we should like to express our grateful thanks to the following:

- Royal College of Nursing for permission to reprint four papers:
  'Labouring in the dark: limitations on the giving of information to enable patients to orientate themselves to the likely events and timescale of labour', by Mavis J. Kirkham, originally published in *Nursing Research: ten studies in patient care*, edited by Jenifer Wilson-Barnett and published in 1983 by John Wiley & Sons.
  'Treatment of depressed women by nurses in Britain and the USA', by Verona Gordon, originally published in *Psychiatric Nursing Research*, edited by Julia Brooking and published in 1986 by John Wiley & Sons.

'Health visitors' and social workers' perceptions of child care problems', by Robert Dingwall and Susan Fox, originally published in *Research in Preventive Community Nursing: fifteen studies in health visiting*, edited by Alison While and published in 1986 by John Wiley & Sons.
'Working with women's health groups: the community health movement', by Jean Orr, also originally published in the collection edited by Alison While.

- John Wiley & Sons for permission to reprint with minor modifications, 'How do women and men in nursing perceive each other?', by George Choon and Suzanne Skevington, originally published in *Understanding Nurses: the social psychology of nursing*, edited by Suzanne Skevington and published in 1984 by John Wiley & Sons.
- Routledge for permission to reprint with minor modifications 'A postscript to nursing' by Nicky James, originally published in *Social Researching: politics, problems, practice*, edited by Colin Bell and Helen Roberts and published in 1984 by Routledge & Kegan Paul.

We are also grateful to Open University Press for permission to re-use 'Leaving it to mum', originally the second part of a longer monograph published in 1987, *Community Care for Mentally Handicapped Children: the origins and consequences of a social policy*.

All of these chapters except the one by Dingwall and Fox (Chapter 9) have been shortened slightly, to enable the 'bones' of the design to emerge clearly. Chapter 8 by Gordon has been further shortened by the excision of material on studies carried out in the USA.

The remaining chapters have not appeared elsewhere in this form. Chapter 6 by Pamela Abbott and Geoff Payne, 'Hospital visiting on two wards', is a shortened version of a research report presented to the Plymouth Community Health Council. Chapter 10 by Abbott *et al.*, 'Health and material deprivation in Plymouth', is a synopsis of *Material Deprivation and Health Status in the Plymouth Health District*, edited by Pamela Abbott and available from the Department of Applied Social Science, Polytechnic South West (Plymouth).

Our approach to social research methods is one of de-mystification. On the whole, research is an extension of what everyone does daily in his or her life. We all look at what is going on about us and draw conclusions from it, and when we want to see what something is like we go and look. When we do not know the answers we ask questions, and we evaluate the information we are given before making use of it. We all have to evaluate our own practice, and very often we come to conclusions about the practice of others. Many of us are in jobs where the evaluation of practice or of information provided by other people is central to our own performance – research in the sense of self-assessment is central to what we do. Many times during our lives we will try out a new way of doing things, or be involved in something new which is imposed on us, and we will form conclusions about its efficacy; that is, we shall want to know if what we are doing works and is an improvement on what went before. All of this can fairly be described as research. What is formally called research differs from it in only three respects.

- First, when formally conducting research we are expected to call on a body of technique and technical expertise. Some of this is indeed difficult – particularly some of the techniques of statistical analysis – but it can be mastered, or if not then we can find others to do it for us; the techniques are not the heart of a research project, but only aids to it.
- Secondly, we are required to be more systematic when formally 'doing research' than we might require of ourselves in coming to private conclusions; the conclusions of formal research must follow logically and cogently from the evidence, and both the conclusions and the evidence are open to public scrutiny.
- Thirdly (and this is the difficult side of researching) a certain attitude or kind of imagination has to be displayed: we have to be vigilant at all times for the possible gaps in our arguments and the possible weaknesses of our procedures.

The book is comprised of three sections. Section A contains three chapters about observation research. Chapter 1 is a participant observation of women in labour and in the pre-labour wards of a hospital, by someone who would be seen by the other participants as a natural member of the setting, even though she declared her role as researcher. She was interested in what information expectant mothers are given and how they obtain and assess information. Chapter 2, by Nicky James, is an extended 'reflexive account' of research which she, a nurse, has carried out on nursing. It demonstrates graphically that research is not a separate thing from the researcher's life – the more so when she does her research in an area which matters to her and in which she already has a role to play. Chapter 3 by Jean Orr gives an account of women's discussion groups for which she acted as convener – a research account of a part of her own professional performance. In each of these three chapters the research is closely related to the practice of the researcher: the first two are studies of nursing and hospital practice by hospital nurses, and the third is by an experienced health visitor assessing the groups she runs as part of her health-education work. The point of the work is not just to gain knowledge, but to modify what is done as a result of what is learned. This kind of research is central to good professional practice.

In Section B we look at ways of asking questions. Chapter 4 is in the 'open' interviewing style – learning about a topic area by getting those involved in it to talk about it in their own way and at their own pace. The research is carried out by 'researchers' rather than practitioners, but with practice-related aims – to provide a basis for evaluating Government policies of community care in the area of mental handicap and to explore the impact of official rhetoric and actions on the lives of carers. Chapter 5 discusses the decisions which have to be made in setting out to administer a more formal questionnaire survey and outlines some of the practical and ethical problems which have to be resolved. Chapter 6 gives the result of one, examining visiting practices in maternity and gynaecology wards by asking the major interested parties – patients, nurses and visitors – a set list of questions ('interview schedule') about the facts of visiting, their attitudes to it and their preferences for change. Again the focus is the effects of a policy change, in this case a change from limited to open visiting on maternity wards which was causing the staff some anxieties. Chapter 7 also collects data on attitudes, but by the more indirect means of semantic differential scale ratings, a psychologist's technique for obtaining standardized responses to stimuli and situations without directly asking for them. The aim in Chapter 7 and other studies like it is to side-step the 'rhetoric' of conscious judgements and reveal 'underlying' action-related beliefs.

Finally, Section C has three chapters included to illustrate the *structure* of a research argument, two of them again closely related to issues of professional practice. Chapter 8 by Verona Gordon, on the treatment of depressed patients by nurses, is a true experiment: a condition is measured beforehand, a treatment is administered to a treatment group and withheld from a comparable 'control group', and the outcome is measured; to the extent that the two groups are indeed comparable, differing only in the fact of participating in the treatment, we may fairly conclude that any differences are due to the treatment. The other two chapters both illustrate how the same logic is applied in circumstances where allocation to treatment and control groups is not possible. Dingwall and Fox in Chapter 9 compare health visitors and social workers as if they were two groups who have received similar treatments (as indeed, do Choon and Skevington in Chapter 7, comparing men and women) and looks for differences between them in their attitudes to the 'child abuse' cases with which both professions may be required to deal. Finally, Chapter 10 by Abbott *et al.*, a 'health and deprivation' study in the tradition of the Black Report (Townsend and Davidson, 1980), stands back from questions of immediate professional practice to look at class and geographical biases in the outcomes of current health policies. It looks for correlation between two variables, but the logic is the same as in the other chapters in Section C – higher levels of an 'explanatory variable' (material deprivation) lead to higher levels of a dependent variable (health status).

One dimension of difference between the papers in this volume is the degree of structure which is imposed on the research situation. The research task ranges from taking notes during group meetings which would have occurred whether or not research was involved (Orr) or recording outcomes of a counselling procedure (Gordon), through note-taking during labour and on labour wards (Kirkham) and tape-recording relatively natural conversations (Abbott and Sapsford), to systematic questionnaire research asking fairly straightforward questions about an easily identifiable phenomenon (Abbott and Payne) or less straightforward ones in a more contrived situation (Choon and Skevington; Dingwall and Fox) to structured re-analysis of records and census information (Abbott *et al.*). The 'measures' used vary from records of natural conversation through direct questions of fact, attitude or belief to complex and indirect psychological 'tests'. Some chapters (e.g. Orr; James) describe just the immediate situation; others survey a difference or a relationship across a population (Choon and Skevington; Dingwall and Fox; Abbott *et al.*); others (Gordon; Abbott and Sapsford) have comparison or control groups to strengthen the logic of their conclusions by excluding some of the other possible explanations of results.

Traditionally in talking about research we make a distinction, in terms of structure, between 'quantitative' and 'qualitatitve' styles of research. Quantitative research, working in the tradition of the physical sciences, aims at reliable measurement of aspects of a situation and seeks to explain variance in these measures – between groups or over time. Its root model is the experiment, described above, with its control group to which treatment is not administered – the argument being that if two groups differ *only* in the treatment they have received, then this treatment must be responsible for any differences between them. Qualitative researchers, on the other hand, are credited with a holistic approach, refusing to dissect the situation into measurable 'variables', and with the kind of attention to naturalism (studying the situation as it really occurs, not as it seems when modified by the research procedures) which would rule out 'treatments' or control groups. To an extent this distinction holds true. As we shall see, however, even qualitative research can be highly structured: Chapter 4 on families of mentally handicapped children has a comparison group which functions very much like a control group, to distinguish what may be attributed to having a family member with learning difficulties from what is 'normal' in all families. The two styles may also not differ drastically in terms of the naturalism of their measurement; it is a moot point whether it is more natural to *contrive* to talk 'naturally' to mothers about their problems (Abbott and Sapsford in Chapter 4, an open interviewing study) or to get people's views by asking questions which are pre-designed but which would seem the natural questions to ask (Abbott and Payne in Chapter 6, a survey).

Questions of representation have also traditionally been associated with 'quantitative' research, and specifically with survey research. The Census asks questions of every member of the population, but most surveys take samples and have to demonstrate that the answers obtained from these samples are typical of what might have been obtained from the population as a whole. On a smaller scale, surveys of particular institutions (e.g. Chapter 6, on visiting practices in one hospital) have to show that the responses they have succeeded in obtaining represent what they would have obtained from asking the questions of every member of the institution, if that had been possible, and they often wish to show also that the institution under investigation is typical of others of its kind. This concern with representation or typicality is in fact general to all styles of research. The experimental treatment of women's depression outlined in Chapter 8 would be of little value if we did not believe that the women who participated in the study were *typical* of the population of women. The studies of male and female nurses, or of social workers and health visitors, are of value only to the extent that we believe the participants were *typical* nurses, health visitors and social workers. The mothers of children with learning difficulties whose views were obtained by 'qualitative' interviewing techniques and are put forward in Chapter 9 are of interest only to the extent that they are *typical* of that group.

We would argue that what unifies all good research is a frame of mind which has been called 'the methodological imagination' (Smith, 1975). Good researchers need to be constantly aware of how participants in the research are making sense of the situation, what it means to them, and also of what it means to the researcher and what he or she may be conditioned to take for granted. This means not just 'collecting data', but long, hard thought about the nature of the situation and the part the researcher plays in shaping and interpreting it, coupled with the realization that the subjects/informants are also interpreting beings and that the sense they make of the situation neces- sarily affects the sense that the researcher can make. This process is called *reflexivity*, and it is not something located in the design stage of a study but continues throughout. (See Chapter 2 for a good example.) What is required is intuitive insight into other people's interpretations, coupled with honesty in examining one's own motives and presuppositions. Qualitative researchers tend to be most conscious of the need for this and to place greater weight on it, but it has an equally important role to play in quantitative research. The other aspect of the methodological imagination is the analytic ability to spot holes in one's own arguments and anticipate possible objections to or alternative explanations of one's results, right from the stage of design. Stress on this tends to be more characteristic of quantitative projects, but it is just as impor- tant in qualitative research to design a project that *is capable in logic* of sus- taining the kinds of conclusions that one may wish to draw. Thus the good researcher is distinguished from the bad one, and from most of us in our 'ordi- nary life' mode of reasoning, by a self-examination, an openness to the experi- ences of others, constant vigilance, a constant questioning of what seems to be occurring, and a constant willingness to be proved wrong. The perfect researcher is therefore an impossible being, someone impossibly self-critical, impossibly far-seeing and impossibly intuitive. However, the researchers represented in this volume have at least *tried* to be good, and there is much to learn from their mistakes and their successes.

Research may be carried out to evaluate one's own professional practice, or to describe and improve the practice of others or of a whole institution. It may explore the shortcomings of current procedures or look to see whether pro- posed new ones are any improvement over what went before. It may be aimed at changing overall policy rather than immediate practice, or be built into the implementation of a change of policy, or be carried out to assess the costs and benefits of a policy change. It may be aimed more generally (e.g. Chapters 7 and 10) at establishing areas of policy where change is desirable and exploring the aspects of policy or customary practice which may be amenable to change – or at adding to the general 'stock of knowledge', which perhaps comes to the same thing. Whatever its aims and its focus, similar concerns and problems underlie all attempts to carry out research systematically, lucidly and usefully.

References

Smith, H.W. (1975). *Strategies of Social Research: the methodological imagination.* Prentice-Hall, New Jersey.

Townsend, P. and Davidson, N. (eds) (1980). *Inequalities in Health.* Penguin, Harmondsworth.

Sapsford, R. and Abbott, P. (1992). *Research Methods for Nurses and the Caring Professions.* Open University Press, Buckingham.

Section A

Observing and participating

Introduction

In this section we present three chapters concerned with investigating research questions by looking at what goes on in a situation in which the researcher is participating. (They are all of the 'qualitative' style; systematic observation, in which one measures the incidence of predetermined behaviours, is discussed in the introduction to Section B.) This is the 'boundary case' between research and everyday experience. The normal way to find out what is going on, or to try out ideas about what is going on, is to go and look for oneself. The major difference between the research stance and that of everyday common sense is that good research is always *disciplined* in a way and to an extent which is seldom (unfortunately) typical of our everyday judgements. The two substantive pieces of research we consider in this section (by Mavis Kirkham and Jean Orr) consist in report of observation: Kirkham observed labour and people's experience of pre-natal wards, and Orr acted as leader for women's self-help discussion groups. The research topics were important for both of them: Kirkham was a trained nurse studying an aspect of hospital practice with the implicit aim of improving it, and Orr was a health visitor looking at some of the many different kinds of 'clients' of health visiting. They do not just claim to report as diarists, however, chronicling 'facts'. They are both properly aware of their impact on the situation and of their intention to 'prove points on the material', and they therefore make every effort to make it equally possible for the opposite to be proved. This is the major discipline of the 'methodological imagination' – to stand far enough back from its own intentions to allow critics the chance to attack them, and to provide the evidence with which they may do so.

The sharpest tool for doing this is *reflexivity* – a process of constantly reflecting on the content and process of the research and trying to be one's own critic. The researcher, while immersed in the social situation, needs at the same time to be very keenly aware of how it would appear to an outsider. He or she needs to be aware of the little things that can determine the nature of the data – interruptions, the presence of outsiders, the injudicious use of a theoretical concept by the researcher herself or himself. Initial introductions are crucial – how the situation is seen by the informants, and therefore what they see as relevant to the researcher, can be determined by the way in which the research is presented by the researcher or, more likely, by the 'gatekeepers' through whom he or she has obtained access to the situation. How the researcher is perceived by the 'real' participants in the situation – as a colleague, a tool of management, a way of influencing management, a snoop, an irrelevant academic – necessarily affects both the access the researcher can gain to the situation and what goes on while he or she is in a position to observe it.

The interpretation of what is going on is further complicated by the fact that the observer is also a participant both in a situation and in the research. We do not record facts in some neutral way, but make sense to ourselves of the sense which participants appear to us to be making of the situation. This means that the *impedimenta* of our previous lives are a part of the research – our attitudes, our social location, our preconceptions. It is necessary to put these by and understand the situation in the way that the participants understand it, but at the same time to maintain distance from the participants and feel free to make a sense of the situation which is *not* necessarily the participants' sense. This is particularly problematic, in terms of feasibility and also in terms of maintaining one's own mental balance, when the situation you are observing is one with which you are thoroughly and professionally familiar and involved. Nicky James' chapter, the second in this section, is an insightful discussion of many of these problems.

Reflexivity appears in two places in the process of research, one visible and one mostly invisible. The visible place for it is in the research report, where the researcher uses reflexive discussion of the research process to demonstrate that his or her conclusions are validly drawn, or to discuss the extent to which validity may be claimed. The invisible but more important place for reflexivity is in the conduct of the research. The methodological imagination requires constant vigilance, constant self-questioning about what may be producing information which is not typical of how the participant might normally speak or behave but be due to something which the researcher has done or some way in which the situation has been presented – *personal reactivity* or *procedural reactivity*. One needs to try to see the situation from the point of view of the participants – the research situation as well as the participants' normal situation – and be sensitively aware of anything which might be influencing what is said or done. The reflexive account in the report is offered as evidence of validity; the reflexive process in the research is what ensures the validity which is reported.

A less emphasized topic in this kind of research, but an important one, is the question of typicality or representative sampling. In a survey asking questions of a sample of some population it would be routine on the part of the researcher to establish to the satisfaction of the reader that the sample is representative of the population, that answers obtained from it are typical of what would be obtained from the whole population. In the smaller-scale and more intense research studies exemplified in this section, however, questions of typicality are equally important. A description of a setting may be thoroughly convincing, but it carries weight only to the extent that we can determine the bounds of generalization. We need to be able to assess whether the situation is unique (and perhaps interesting, but of no importance outside its own confines), or typical of certain extremes, or typical of the 'middle range' of a whole class of similar situations which might include ones which we ourselves will probably encounter. Mavis Kirkham's chapter would be less interesting if we thought that the cases she observed and the handling of information were specific to the hospital in which she observed them, rather than typical of maternity cases and maternity wards. Jean Orr's chapter would be read differently if we supposed that she was describing two unique groups and that what she said had no bearing whatsoever on groups which we ourselves might join or run.

## 1

Labouring in the dark: Limitations on the giving of information to enable patients to orientate themselves to the likely events and timescale of labour

Mavis Kirkham

Today almost all women in this country experience labour as patients. Often this is their first experience of hospitalization though antenatal care may serve as a training in the patient role (Graham, 1977). They therefore need to adjust both to being patients and to the technical setting of the labour ward.

Technical developments have made possible accurate monitoring and adjustment of the physiological variables of labour. Though the general usefulness of obstetric innovation is much debated, the equipment involved highlights the abnormal and thereby may contribute to the security of staff and patients. The connections to the various machines involved plus the convenience of the staff greatly limit the patient's physical movement and decrease her comfort. Analgesic technology has, however, advanced at a great pace. Epidural anaesthesia has revolutionized pain relief in labour. Yet whilst removing pain it also removes sensation from the area concerned which can further emphasize the patient's passive role. Experiencing discomfort caused by her setting, yet lacking pain and also feedback from her body, the patient has considerable need for information and is better able to absorb it than a patient in pain. Being in an unfamiliar setting and in the care of strangers greatly increases the information she seeks.

There are problems in the transmission of information within any institutional setting. Riley (1977) looked at the structural organization of maternity hospitals in this light:

The best-informed reforms will not succeed in making hospitals fully humane, since institutions which depend on rigidly maintained

hierarchy and strict division of labour among their personnel cannot fail
to transfer the results in some form to the treatment of patients . . . the
difficulties of acquiring a theoretical appreciation of need are as nothing
compared with the difficulties of *enacting* flexibility within an inflexibly
organised system.

The very reasons for the existence of hospitals; the centralization of medical
expertise and equipment for maximum efficiency, to a large extent dictate the
structure and, therefore, the problems of the patients within that structure.
Freidson (1970) looked at the implications of the professional dominance
caused by medical expertise;

> . . . the dominant profession stands in an entirely different structural
> relationship to the division of labour than does the subordinate profes-
> sion. In essence, the difference reflects the existence of a *hierarchy of
> institutional expertise* . . . [which] can have the same effect upon the
> experience of the client as bureaucracy is said to have.

Many studies have shown that communication with hospital patients is generally inadequate (McGhee, 1961; Raphael, 1969; Franklin, 1974). Various
reasons have been suggested for staff's failure to give information to patients.
These include a view amongst staff that talking to patients is a waste of
precious time, the need of the staff to limit their involvement with patients as a
defence against anxiety (Barnes, 1961) and doctors' tendency to underrate
those aspects of nursing care which cannot be measured scientifically (*Lancet*,
1970). Another factor is the way in which patients internalize these very
pressures. As Tagliacozzo and Mauksch (1979) observed; '"good patients"
withdraw from those on whom they depend and with whom they wish to
communicate but whom they do not wish "to bother"'.

Such a situation is documented in hospitals caring for the sick. The changes
in maternity care have brought normal birth within this model. The recognition of the midwife as a limited practitioner (Midwives Act, 1902) was only
possible within the limits set by the medical profession as to the extent of her
responsibilities and training (Cope, 1959). This left her, within the limits set
down in the Act, as an independent practitioner in cases of normal childbirth.
As normal birth moved into hospital, the doctors' field, definitions changed.
Previously, all pregnancies were seen as normal until judged otherwise, a
judgement usually made initially by the midwife. The reverse is now true as all
pregnancies fall under medical management and are 'normal only in retro-
spect' (Percival, 1970). By this logic the midwife as a practitioner in her own
right is defined out of existence, and the hospital midwives' work during
labour is either obstetric nursing or what medical staff define as provisionally
normal and are therefore prepared to delegate.

Within such a structure the position of the midwife, despite our cherished
legal and professional definition, clearly parallels that of the nurse. There has
been little research on midwives and the giving of information but there has
been considerable research on nurses in this respect. Manikheim (1979)
observed:

Patterns of communication between nurses and patients reflect this authority/subordinate role. The care recipient has been a passive, dependent model. It has been relatively easy for nurses, having been conditioned as women, to relate to the passive model and to discourage independence and autonomy in clients. The nurse often evades direct questions from the patient. . . . This communication style indirectly negates the nurse's understanding of the patient's condition from the patient's perspective.

Faulkner (1980) described student nurses 'saying nothing to be safe' and ignoring patients' cues. Macleod Clark (1981) described the strategies nurses use to control conversation – avoiding issues raised by patients, blocking talk and using stereotyped patterns of conversation as well as ignoring cues offered by patients who felt unable to ask direct questions. Johnston (1976) found nurses inadequate in assessing the type of information patients required.

Whilst nursing in the USA is different in many ways from British nursing, Sheahan's (1972) stark analysis of the effects of the hospital power structure on American nursing is of relevance. She saw doctors' professional decisions as determining the care of hospital patients and therefore the roles of those who contribute to that care. Power rests with the doctor rather than the nurse and she concludes: 'If power corrupts, so much more so does powerlessness. It corrupts by changing our perceptions of ourselves . . . being too subordinate, too alienated or too weak to effect change.' If nursing is thus constrained by the hospital structure it seems highly unlikely that nurses will feel able to give information to patients which may give patients a potential for decision-making.

Despite this dilemma fundamental to hospital nursing, communication is widely seen as a basic component of nursing (e.g. MacFarlane, 1980). The structure which gives rise to the nurse's dilemma also increases the patient's need for information. They need explanations about what is happening (Barnes, 1961) and need to become familiar with their new setting (Franklin, 1974), as well as seeking information about their illness, treatment and progress.

When systematic attempts are made to give information, the results are striking. Research has shown the good effects of giving pre-operative information on post-operative pain and all aspects of recovery (Hayward, 1975; Boore, 1978). A small study has shown improved nurse–patient communication can very rapidly reduce patients' pain and decrease use of analgesics (Tarasuk et al., 1965). Another American study showed similar pain relief resulting from nurse information-giving linked to patient decision-making (Moss and Meyer, 1966).

Such research is clearly of relevance to midwives working with patients in labour in hospital. The woman in labour is well and undertaking one of the most strenuous tasks of her life. She needs to orientate herself to her labour and to her setting as well as to cope with pain. If she labours in a single room she cannot learn from her peers as most hospital patients do, so she is completely dependent upon the staff for information. Her brief period of patienthood is also a rite of passage since labour is the physiological introduction to parenthood. Is a labour spent as a passive patient lacking the information necessary even for orientation an appropriate introduction to the activity and responsibility of parenthood? Though the hospital midwife experiences the same dilemmas basic to her role and setting as does the nurse, she is the person to whom the woman in labour looks for the information she seeks. . . .

Studies of maternity services such as those by Cartwright (1979) and Oakley (1980) were conducted retrospectively by interviews. The consistency of their results led me to believe that there was now a need for a different approach. I therefore wanted to see what it was that actually happened during the course of labour which was likely to lead to results of the kind so consistently found in research conducted by means of interviews.

Method

I wanted to see what issues were important to those involved as shown in their actions and words at the time. Observation was clearly the appropriate method. Labour is a definite process which can be observed.

Participant observation (Becker, 1970) was chosen as a method of observation which imposed the minimum of external structure upon observations. Ethnographic interviews (Spradly, 1979) were used to help place in context the data gained by observation.

I came to this research as a midwife and a mother. But my observations were guided by those aspects of care in labour which the midwives and mothers I observed showed were important to them. Thus my observations and analysis were 'grounded' (Glaser and Strauss, 1967) in the experience of those observed as shown in their words and actions.

I sat during most of the labours level with the patient's head about six feet from her and took constant written notes. The question of the researcher's influence upon the research is raised by this method. It arises at all levels of observation and analysis for as Hanson (1958), the philosopher of science, observed: 'People, not their eyes, see. Cameras and eyeballs are blind.'

Though my role was that of observer, I participated in conversation initiated by those I observed. This was of importance in building relationships with them and yielded much useful information.

The people I observed may well have been on their 'best behaviour' because I was observing them. This, in itself, highlights what behaviour is seen as 'best'. The people I observed had more important pressures upon them than those caused by my presence and these were the things I wanted to study. Thus the opportunity to study these pressures at work, plus the relative insignificance they give to the observer, together, make up the great advantage of the method.

This paper is based upon observations taken down in writing during ninety labours in a consultant unit in a teaching hospital in a northern city. The women whose labours I observed were also interviewed post-natally. Eighty-five patients in the same unit were interviewed ante-natally. I also observed five home confinements in the same city and eighteen labours in a GP Unit in an adjacent rural area. Many of the midwives concerned were interviewed at the end of the fieldwork.

These labours were chosen as normal labours, as far as anyone can tell this in advance. I therefore did not observe women with known medical or obstetrical abnormalities. Nor did I observe where care may have been unusual, for example private patients or staff.

This is a piece of qualitative, descriptive research which does not aim to be statistical.

Findings

The patient's search for information

. . .

All the patients I interviewed wanted information with which to orientate themselves and described their ideal midwife as one who volunteered such information. Mrs 56 said: 'If they don't tell you, you don't know where you are.' I was repeatedly told: 'You need to know'; 'You need to know or you're in the dark'; 'To know what to expect'; 'To know so you're prepared'; 'To know so you're not frightened'; 'As long as I know what's going on I'm O.K.' For many women the main thing they wanted of the midwife was for her: 'To constantly tell you exactly what's happening all the time' (Mrs 73). The word 'exactly' was very frequently used in this context.

Some women conceded that 'there are women who don't want to know', but no-one included herself in this category. Many women expressed the need 'not to be fobbed off' or said they wanted 'honest answers not the brushoff'. They acknowledged the uncertainties of labour and wanted the midwife to share her estimates, 'even if she's wrong' and especially if labour did not progress normally. 'I'd rather know than just look at their faces', said Mrs 55. 'I was a bit at a loss. Then she said "If the head doesn't turn you'll need forceps." I was glad she said that. I was prepared.' said Mrs 20. All the women I interviewed wanted to be 'prepared' in this sense.

Patients in other hospital settings gain information from their peers (Roth, 1963). The woman in labour, lacking this source of information, is in this respect, as in many others, particularly dependent upon the staff. The staff are important to her and she is considerate towards them.

In order to be considerate she has first to learn the values of the staff. She therefore shows respect for their expertise and learns staff priorities from their actions and the cues they give.

The admission procedure is in this sense highly educational for the patient. The form-filling usually starts with: 'When did your contractions become regular?' Patients' replies to this question are often quite lengthy descriptions of the circumstances and sensations of early labour. The form requires a short precise answer and the midwife usually fills it in with a remark such as: 'I'll put 4.30.' After that the patients' replies typically become much shorter. Similarly if, after examining the patient, the midwife tells her something of her findings, the patient is likely to ask one or more questions which will put this information into context for herself. If she is told nothing she usually feels she should not ask. The patients I observed were very eager to please and to do the 'right thing'. But their need for information remained.

Patients of higher social class convey to the staff an image of themselves as articulate and clearly used to obtaining information and taking decisions. Their social skills and general manner create an atmosphere in which staff are likely to give information. A student midwife said to Mrs 13 (librarian, married to a company director, ex-city councillor): 'I assess my patients by their intelligence and see what they will understand. Like you can see that monitor's not working.' Several patients of lower social class in the same situation thought the baby's heart had stopped when there was no trace on the monitor but did not like to ask about it.

Patients of social class 1 or 2 (by the Registrar General's Classification), because they will 'understand', are offered more information without asking questions. For instance Mrs 54 (a social worker married to a vet) was told by sister in early labour that a vaginal examination was necessary before pain relief could be given 'so bear in mind that it will take about 20 minutes'. Staff also tended to ask such patients about their perceptions and preferences during labour. Such conversation made it possible for these patients to make decisions and exercise choice.

Patients of lower social class or less 'intelligence' did not receive more information to balance their lack, though my interviews with them showed that they wanted it. They were given sparse information apparently because they were felt to be less likely to 'understand'. Staff seemed to find such patients less predictable or trustworthy within the setting of the ward. The emotional order of this setting was a source of security for the staff which they did not wish disturbed. They were, therefore, unlikely to entrust patients with information unless the patients could in some way set the staff at ease and establish themselves as trustworthy in their eyes. Various tactics were used to achieve this.

Tactics for gaining information

Questions

Questions are the obvious way to gather information. On the labour ward this is not easy. For a question to be asked someone has to make themselves available to answer the question. Patients are likely to ask questions if:

1. The person they are asking has been present for a few minutes and appears likely to stay long enough to answer the question.
2. That person is sitting near the patient rather than standing over her or at a great distance from her.

3. That person is not speaking herself.
4. That person is looking at the patient, rather than the notes, the monitor or a colleague.
5. That person is not actually causing pain or discomfort to the patient at the time (e.g. by doing a vaginal examination or putting up a drip).

These criteria are unlikely to be met on precisely those occasions when the staff learn new information about the progress of the labour (such as vaginal examination). They are also least likely to be met by those staff (obstetricians and sisters) who take decisions about the course of the labour. Patients 'don't like to ask' such people (unless they make themselves available for questioning), because they feel they are 'interrupting' them, as they are clearly 'busy'.

Patients are frequently left feeling unable to approach the senior staff, who hold information, out of respect. On the other hand, the junior staff (such as student midwives) who sit with patients and are approachable either do not hold the information or feel unable to give it, so patients stop asking them out of sympathy with their situation.

If early questions are answered, the patient feels able to ask further questions. If early questions are deflected or blocked the patient soon feels she should not ask questions and stops. Early questions may also be ignored. An unanswered question is socially uncomfortable and unlikely to be repeated.

For the vast majority of patients there are few occasions when they feel they can ask questions and a general feeling that they should not. Many patients said to me post-natally: 'If I'd asked they might have said. But you don't like to ask.' For such women other strategies are needed.

Statements

Statements have an advantage over questions in that a midwife may take up a statement and given information but a statement does not have to be answered. If there is no response no-one feels uncomfortable so the patient feels able to try again, for example, Mrs 75 after delivery:

    1.37 P: My bottom feels sore. I suppose it's where they cut. [Silence]
    1.42 P: My backside's hurting. It'll be the cut. [Silence]
    1.46 P: [Winces] It's the episiotomy.
           S: It's not an episiotomy. It's a tear. But it hasn't gone anywhere it shouldn't. I didn't have time to get the instruments out let alone cut.

Statements may also work where questions fail. By the reaction of staff to statements about her feelings a patient can also learn what is appropriate and possible and thus what can be asked.

Jokes

Jokes, like statements, can be used as direct conversational tactics where questions fail to glean the required information. For example, Mrs 72 after artificial rupture of membranes:

P: Is there much water?
Dr: A normal amount.
P: You imagine buckets.
Dr: You've not got that much when you get to term, gets less after 38 weeks and more will be held back by the baby's head.

Similarly a remark by a patient to her husband such as, 'you'll be out of here in time to wet the baby's head', may lead the midwife to estimate the likely time of delivery in relation to the pub's closing time. As well as gleaning specific information, humour can create a relaxed atmosphere conducive to the giving of information on subjects unrelated to those joked about.

Patients' jokes almost always concerned themselves or their husbands. They were laughing at themselves and encouraging the staff to laugh with them. They were not laughing at the staff or the setting. Thus their humour emphasized their humble role and their acceptance of it. This joking visibly increased the ease of the staff. This was shown in increased conversation with the patient, more smiles and more eye contact with her. Patients who joked were entrusted with more information than most patients I observed. Most of these patients were of social class 3.

Most patients, even of social class 3, did not joke. Joking was done more by husbands or by husband and wife teams than by patients alone. Some strategies were confined to patients.

Self-denigration

Some women appeared to use self-denigration to make clear that their view of themselves, and their search for information, was meant as no threat to the staff. Fat women were often very skilled at this. For example Mrs 21 (part of a long sequence of self-denigration initiated by the patient).

[*The fetal heart monitor is not working*]
Student Midwife: Let's see if this machine is playing silly beggars.
P: [Pulls up her gown to show the wire and its connection to the monitor]
SM: You're a right flasher aren't you?
P: And I've got such a wonderful body.
[Both laugh]
SM: [Listens to fetal heart]
P: [Asks if she can listen]
SM: [Lets her listen with a stethoscope]
SM: [Takes patient's blood pressure] It's fine now, your BP.
[*It was high earlier*]

Other patients had similar tactics of self-denigration in repeatedly referring to themselves as 'a baby' or 'a terrible coward'. Staff varied in the amount of information they gave but always treated these patients sympathetically and information-seeking remarks, linked to self-denigration, were not ignored. Clearly such techniques are not only used in labour, and their development and use await analysis.

Eavesdropping

One of the main ways patients in this hospital gained information about the likely course of the rest of their labours was by listening to the sisters teaching student midwives or medical students. Indeed Mrs 41 said that she had taken an Open University course between her first and second labours to enable her to understand the technical terms involved in this teaching.

This teaching took place over the patient's abdomen (indeed sister often kept her hand on the patient's abdomen throughout) but did not include her. Some patients were told: 'This doesn't concern you.' A few patients (all social class 1 or 2) were specifically included in teaching sessions and invited to ask questions. For the vast majority this was not so.

This teaching could help meet the patient's need for information as to likely eventualities, as well as to the likely timescale of the labour. But because the patient is eavesdropping she is not in a position to ask for what she learns to be put in context. For example, Mrs 65 observed post-natally 'I picked up the result of the examination from the teaching. But I didn't know how many centimetres there were.' (That is, in full dilatation of the cervix, so she did not know how far she still had to go.) Furthermore some patients were really frightened when sister took the educational opportunity to generalize from her case to abnormalities which were unlikely in this labour.

The passivity of this method of gaining information lay at the heart of both its advantages and disadvantages. All patients used it because it was available to them without causing any inconvenience to staff. But it was not designed to meet their needs and could be frightening.

Watching and drawing conclusions

This is in many ways the visual equivalent of eavesdropping. This was used, particularly, to try to work out the likely timescale of a labour. For example:

Mrs 15: If it was going to be quick they wouldn't have given me the Pethidine.

Mrs 8: They can't think I'm progressing because they brought me tea.

As with eavesdropping the information is useful only if the patient can place it in the right context.

The move to the delivery room was an example often seen differently by patients and staff. In this hospital, patients were put in a delivery room at 3 cm cervical dilatation or earlier. Some patients, when put in the room in which

they would deliver, thought that the delivery was imminent and became
increasingly disappointed as it became clear that this was not so. As Mrs 65
said later: 'I felt ignorant because I felt I would deliver soon after getting to the
delivery room. I didn't know how long it would go on. I kept thinking I was
going to deliver soon. I would have appreciated some kind of estimate.' It was
clear that Mrs 65 felt her ignorance as a reprehensible state akin to stupidity,
not something she could remedy by asking staff for information though she
'would have appreciated' this.

Language

Patients in labour do not have their own language or culture to which they
belong. Conversation between staff and patients takes place in language
chosen by the staff even if this is a matter of the staff choosing lay terms. For
example:

P: I've got a pain in my, er.
M: Your bottom?
P: I've got a pain in my bottom.

Such exchanges were very common.
   In adopting the language of the ward the patient also adopts its values.

[Mrs 15 is with her husband. She appears very relaxed during contractions but becomes anxious to know how her labour is progressing. After
some debate she rings the bell. Nursing auxiliary answers the bell]
P: Can you judge how far on I am? . . .
NA: Oh. You're distressed. [Leaves]

The patient has learnt the language of the ward and the legitimate reason for
ringing the bell. When sister arrives she refers to herself as 'distressed' and her
distress is relieved by an injection. In adopting the language of 'distress', and
thus doing what the staff expected of her, Mrs 15 stopped asking questions
and did not learn 'how far on' she was until she delivered.
   The language of the labour ward is the language of obstetrics which measures the objective progress, or otherwise, of the labour. Such measurements
are not usually given to the patient. There is no language, here, to describe the
patient's perceptions of labour. In expressing, or simply experiencing the
labour subjectively she is, therefore, likely to feel at odds with her attendants
whom she seeks to please. When this is so she apologizes.
   Most of the patients I observed apologized during labour. Many apologized
frequently if they felt they were not behaving well or were 'being a nuisance' or
'causing trouble' by making requests or simply receiving routine care from
staff who were busy. The commonest words I heard patients say immediately
after delivery were, 'I'm sorry', usually addressed to the midwife. Clearly the
habit of apology comes from life outside the labour ward. Nevertheless, to use
it here the patient must accept an external standard of behaviour, that of the
staff, against which she judges herself to be inadequate. Staff find apology

acceptable. As the anthropologist and linguist Sapir said in 1928: 'Language is a guide to social reality. . . . Human beings . . . are very much at the mercy of the particular language which has become the medium of expression of their society.' The patients, 'at the mercy of the particular language' of the labour ward can only apologize. The language reflects and legitimates the power structure of the setting.

Limitations on midwives' information-giving

The importance of giving information was stressed by most of the midwives I interviewed. Their words echoed those patients used in describing their desire for information and showed considerable uniformity and perceptiveness. 'Explain'; 'Explain everything you do'; 'Don't leave her in the dark'; 'Keep them informed'; 'Explain the doctor's action'; 'Say what you're going to do before you do it'; 'Give information to allay fear'; 'Give honest explanations'; 'Don't fob her off.' These things were said to be repeatedly both as what the midwives felt were important aspects of their work and what they felt patients wanted of them. In this context many of them went on to stress that 'everyone is different' so it is important to 'explain at her level'. In practice there are many constraints on the midwife's explanations.

As the patient's conversation is tailored to what the staff find acceptable, so the staff seek in their conversation to please colleagues senior to themselves. The assumed priorities of senior staff, therefore, considerably affect the speech and action of those more junior staff who spend most time with patients.

The presence of senior staff greatly inhibits the giving of information to patients. I repeatedly saw sister explain a doctor's decisions to a patient immediately after the doctor left the room. Likewise, student midwives would explain the results of an examination immediately after the sister left the room. I did not observe any student midwife being told to give information to a patient or being criticized for not giving it. In this sense the junior staff's assessment of the priorities of their senior colleagues appears to be accurate. Indeed it seems to be considered wiser to omit the giving of information as a precaution against saying the wrong thing. Staff therefore learn to block or deflect patients' attempts to gain information.

P: How long does it take?
S: Babies come when they're ready. [Changes subject]

or

P: [*In early labour*] I don't know what to expect.
SM: You don't with your first.
[End of conversation]

The patient thereby learns not to ask.

Feeling unable to give information, midwives often give reassurance. Remarks such as: 'Don't worry'; 'We're very on the ball here'; 'You're in the right place' are very common in moments of anxiety and are often given in response to direct questions from the patient. Books on communication condemn such techniques, for example Burton (1958), 'reassurance is belittling to the person who has the problem or worry. . . . An immediate effect of this response is to block the person from expressing further feeling'. This blocking technique has the further sophistication that it appears to make the midwife feel better.

Midwives seem attached to routines. (Perhaps they make us feel secure?) Although many routine tasks are clearly of more importance than information giving, midwives still want to give information so they often develop their own routine patter for this. Such information tends to be compressed into packages beginning: 'What we'll do is. . .'. These routine packages, whilst they are easy for the midwife to deliver, may not be easy for the patient to digest. Such patter usually concerns procedures which, lacking feedback, are described from the midwives' viewpoint. So points of great concern to individual patients are omitted and the patient 'does not like to ask'.

Other settings

Conversation in labour differed considerably in the different settings I observed.

In the GP Unit, without medical staff, students or inexperienced midwives, the midwives worked as equals on their own territory. They had no senior colleagues to inhibit their conversation with patients. Furthermore, lacking technical advances in pain relief, they had to gain the patient's co-operation by attention to her physical and mental comfort. Conversation and information-giving reflected this. Patients of all social classes were given more information. (They also experienced more pain.) Patients in the GP Unit sought to please the staff but their behaviour could show wider differences than in the consultant unit, and still be acceptable.

Patients at home were on their own territory. They did not use humble techniques for gaining information. (Apologies were mainly addressed to husbands.) Midwives in the patient's home lack colleagues and their relationship with their patient was in many ways colleague-like. These midwives gave much more information. They often gave a running commentary on their actions in advance. Thus the patient was able to refuse a procedure and some did, which was not seen in hospital. Patient behaviour was tailored to standards which she had chosen before the labour and the midwife was informed of this by the patient and her husband. This provided a sharp contrast with the hospital patient's great efforts to conform to the standards of the institution which she had to learn by observation and humility.

Concluding thoughts and hopes

The patients I observed wanted information with which to orientate themselves to their labours and the midwives wanted to give information. Yet despite considerable efforts on both sides the information given was usually inadequate especially for those women whose need was greatest.

In conforming to the standards of the ward most patients sought information in passive ways which could not gather information specific to their needs. Midwives gave information when ward circumstances permitted, which usually excluded just those occasions when information was learned or decisions taken. These were also the occasions when the patient was most anxious to know what was happening.

Lack of information prevents the possibility of patients exercising choice. This may be convenient for staff within an institution but makes it impossible to respond to patient's individual needs, which the midwives I interviewed wanted to do. Passive patients do not 'trouble' the smooth running of the ward but this is hardly a healthy state (Seligman, 1975) or a good preparation for parenthood. In this sense it goes against the basic aims of midwifery.

In the strategies they use to gain or give information without 'causing trouble' to the basic order of the ward, there are striking parallels between the actions of patients and midwives. These tactics are not unique to labour but are developed over a lifetime, or career, as ways of coping from an inferior position. Patient apologizes to midwife, junior midwife apologizes to sister, sister apologizes to doctor. Similarly, each observes and learns by indirect means rather than asking questions and thus confessing 'ignorance' and risking discomfort if unanswered. Midwives, as much as patients, lack an appropriate language and in adopting the language of obstetrics, adopt too its values and its limitations. Yet it is these very limitations which ensure the continuation of midwifery.

I believe that an awareness of these parallels alone could do much to change communication patterns in midwifery. The midwife is still 'with woman' in the very words she utters just where that woman's needs are met the least. An awareness of this would not threaten the life-saving scientific progress enshrined in our hospitals but would enable the midwife to 'dissect the fat from the muscle in the imputed skill of the professional service worker and to determine the consequences of each for what is done to the client, with what price' (Freidson, 1970).

The midwife's information-giving can change the patient's experience of her labour whatever the setting:

Mrs 70:   I don't think pain is half so bad if you know how long it's for.

Mrs 39:   I still felt in control, although I couldn't feel anything, because she stayed and told me what was happening and helped me move. So it was as if I'd got my legs. [*With epidural*]

Mrs 61:   I didn't know. I had no sense of where I was. No light at the end of the tunnel. It seems infinite and it weighs on your mind very heavily.

The midwife can provide this 'light'. She cannot do this as an individual in the face of institutional pressures. If supported by the priorities of her profession and the emphasis of her education, however, she may be able to give the information her patients seek.

References

Barnes, E. (1961). *People in Hospitals*. Macmillan, London.
Becker, H. S. (1970). *Sociological Work*. Aldine, Chicago.
Boore, J. R. P. (1978). *Prescription for Recovery*. Royal College of Nursing, London.
Burton, G. (1958). *Personal, Impersonal and Interpersonal Relations*. Springer, New York.
Cartwright, A. (1979). *The Dignity of Labour?* Tavistock, London.
Classification of Occupations (1970). HMSO, London.
Cope, Z. (1959). 'The licence in midwifery in the Royal College of Surgeons', in *The Royal College of Surgeons of England: A History*, Chapter 15. Blunt, London.
Faulkner, A. (1980). Communication and the nurse. *Nursing Times*, Occasional Paper, Sept. 4, 93–95.
Franklin, B. (1974). *Patient Anxiety on Admission to Hospital*. Royal College of Nursing, London.
Freidson, E. (1970). *Professional Dominance: The Social Structure of Medical Care*. Aldine, Chicago.
Glaser, B. and Strauss, A. L. (1967). *The Discovery of Grounded Theory*. Aldine, Chicago.
Graham, H. (1977). 'Womens' attitudes to conception and pregnancy', in *Equalities and Inequalities in Family Life* (eds R. Chester and J. Peel). Academic Press, London.
Hanson N. R. (1958). *Patterns of Discovery*. Cambridge University Press, New York.
Hayward, J. (1975). *Information – A Prescription Against Pain*. Royal College of Nursing, London.
Johnston, M. (1976). 'Communication of patients feelings in hospital', in *Communication Between Doctors and Patients* (ed. A. E. Bennett). Oxford University Press for the Nuffield Provincial Hospitals Trust, Oxford.
Lancet (1970). Doctor and Nurse. *Lancet*, 2(7680), 971–972.
Macleod Clark, J. (1981). Communication in nursing. *Nursing Times*, 77(1), 12–18.
McFarlane of Llandaff (1980). Preface to P. Ashworth. *Care to Communicate*. Royal College of Nursing, London.
McGhee, A. (1961). *The Patient's Attitude to Nursing Care*. Livingstone, London.
Manikheim, M. L. (1979). 'Communication patterns of women and nurses', in *Women in Stress: A Nursing Perspective* (eds D. L. Kjevick and I. M. Martinson). Appleton-Century-Crofts, New York.
The Midwives Act (1902). 2EDW7C17. HMSO, London.
Ministry of Health (1959). *Report of a Maternity Services Committee* (Cranbrook Report). HMSO, London.
Moss, F. T. and Meyer, B. (1966). The effects of nursing interaction upon pain relief in patients. *Nursing Research*, 15(4), 303–306.
Oakley, A. (1980). *Women Confined: Towards a Sociology of Childbirth*. Martin Robertson, Oxford.
Percival, R. (1970). Management of normal labour. *The Practitioner*, No. 1221, 204, March.
Raphael, W. (1969). *Patients and their Hospitals*. King Edward's Hospital Fund for London, London.
Report on Investigation into Maternal Mortality (1937). HMSO, London.

Riley, E. M. D. (1977). 'What do women want? – The question of choice in the conduct of labour', in *Benefits and Hazards of the New Obstetrics* (eds T. Chard and
M. Richards). Spastics International Medical Publications. Heinemann, London.

Roth, J. (1963). *Timetables: Structuring the Passage of Time in Hospital Treatment
and Other Careers*. Bobbs-Merrill, New York.

Sapir, E. (1928). *Culture, Language and Personality* (1966 edition, edited by
D. G. Mandelbaum). University of California Press, Berkley.

Seligman, M. E. P. (1975). *Helplessness: On Depression, Development and Death*.
Friedman, San Francisco.

Sheahan, D. (1972). The game of the name: nurse professional and nurse technician.
Nursing Outlook, 20(7), July, 440–444.

Spradley, J. P. (1979). *The Ethnographic Interview*. Holt, Rinehart and Winston,
New York.

Tagliacozzo, D. L. and Mauksch, H. O. (1979). 'The patient's view of the patient's
role', in *Patients, Physicians and Illness* (eds E. G. Jaco). The Free Press, New
York.

Tarasuk, M. B., Rhymes, J. and Leonard, R. C. (1965). 'An experimental test of the
importance of communication skills for effective nursing', in *Social Interaction
and Patient Care* (eds J. K. Skipper and R. C. Leonard). J. B. Lippincott,
Philadelphia.

## 2

A postscript to nursing

Nicky James

Nicky, you're sort of like a P.S. in a letter. Not part of the main body of
the nursing team, but still important.

> Night nurse at the hospital

This is our pet sociologist who's working on the unit and studying us.
She's found out all sorts of interesting things.

> Continuing care unit Sister, introducing me to an outsider.

. . .

Narrowing down the task

Not knowing how the research system worked granted me the luxury of submitting, unperturbed, an outline, both vague and short, which managed to
supply me with a department from which to work, and an initial two years'
money from a central fund, with the possibility of a third year. The department was where I had done my undergraduate degree, and the mixed blessings
of familiarity saved at least some of the groundwork of establishing myself.
My supervisor, a vital ingredient whose importance I had not recognized, had
overseen the undergraduate dissertation from which the postgraduate study
was to develop. We agreed with minimal discussion to continue with each
other. Approachable and non-directive as he was, he left me to discover a
problem that interested me from reading which included spiritualism, psycho-
analysis, census data, ethics, medicine, government reports, and so on. Some-
how from this bewildering wealth, a question had to be chosen that could be
followed up to reach some kind of conclusion. The distractions of philosophy
held no more appeal than the abstractions of grand theory, so it was fortuitous
that I was able to build on the tensions I found between being an academic and
being a nurse.

Nurses *do* things as their work. . . . If they are not doing something physical
they are not working, and to be in a sociology department concentrating on
the written word and discussion seemed egocentric and indulgent. Thus one of

the easiest decisions on how to solidify the nebulous thesis was to make it empirical, using previous knowledge. Such a decision had a huge impact, far from clear at the time, because it not only structured the projected three years into a manageable timetable, but to me implied a particular way of thinking, which excluded number crunching and hypothesis testing – both, then, sociology of derision. Thinking in terms of interpersonal relations, I wanted to know how people affected each other in looking after the dying (which at the time I took to be a passive event for the patient) and where the power of decision lay.

Interwined with considering more specifically what I wanted to do was the input from others. During the initial weeks I discovered there were different groups of people relevant to the project – outsiders, university staff, other postgraduates and friends. Needless to say, these shifted categories over time. I also worked on the basis that there were two types of problems, acceptable ones you feel you can ask about and unacceptable ones which are more difficult to ask and which are matched more carefully against the audience.

The staff, whom I already knew, although unclear on the resources available for postgraduates . . . were a source of endless suggestions of people to see and expansive lists of books and articles to read. Knowing that they could not all be seen or read, it was difficult to evaluate which to choose. To optimize their preferred help required knowing what I was doing at the very time I was least sure.

The list of references grew alarmingly in inverse proportion to the clarity of the problem. Some friends were intrigued enough to be useful sounding boards, asking questions which, in encouraging me to explain simply, helped sort the irrelevant from the necessary to the enlightening. Others were part of the network keeping me informed of radio and television programmes, talks and newspaper articles, also providing light entertainment when the dark side of death was looming large.

In January, four months after starting, I attended a multidisciplinary terminal care course with nurses, social workers, clergy and a few doctors. From taking embarrassingly more notes than anyone else, and feeling like neither nurse nor researcher, it occurred to me that spoken repetition on the course of written phrases in the literature, which encapsulate 'good' terminal care, such as 'teamwork', 'individual patient assessment', 'death with dignity', could be used as categories of observation. Sociologically this carried all the dangers of using language generated within and by the groups being observed, but they were of value because commendable as ideals, though I thought there might be some obstacles to their practice. They also served the useful function of giving credibility to a study within the medical settings in which I thought it might be pertinent to work.

A few weeks later when 'The role of the nurse in the care of the dying' had been achieved as the working title, I began to formulate the kind of fieldwork I was going to do, and devise ways of becoming acceptable to nursing administrators – hoping to use the sway of past nursing training. So 'staff' spread from academics to National Health administrators.

Despite the profoundly good advice of an anthropologist who told me that projects should be limited to take home life into account, it took a formal discussion with three nursing hierarchs to alter my grandiose schemes. The meeting was a fascinating struggle between my two roles of nurse and researcher, with the former winning. Although medical sociology was well established locally, I had thought that being introduced so officially to people I wanted to work with on the wards might make me a threat. Instead, using old nursing contacts, I made my own way.

In the proposal to the nursing administrators, submitted before I went to see them, I tried to 'sell' myself by predicting what they would like, and also what they would dislike, so that it could be counteracted. The proposal was deliberately left flexible so that there was room for manoeuvre, but my main doubt was that they would tolerate an observer. Why should they? To try to overcome that, I made a commitment to working free, instead of being an onlooker, and the more I thought about it the more I thought it would provoke interesting data. . . .

As it was I totally misjudged their reading of the proposal. Instead of being flexible it looked as though I did not know what I was doing, and though they welcomed nursing research, there was some anxiety over someone who wanted to be integrated. The effectiveness that the authority of nursing administrators can have on those they train showed, and I acquiesced to their suggestions that I drop totally the community part of a scheme which had included time to be spent in a community, in a hospital, and in a hospice.

In the report on the meeting I noted that 'I went in optimistic and came out feeling like a grilled sardine – small, squashed and hot'.

Having given me their tentative support, the administrators continued to meet me intermittently, and they helped devise the proposal to go before the Ethical Committee. At the time it caused enormous concern since the project could be stopped, but once it was accepted the whole thing vanished as unimportant, with the exception that they made me have a nurse supervisor. A senior tutor at the Infirmary Nursing School, she not only let me talk at her, but eased my way into the nursing school, allowing me freely to use the library and video facilities, and by the end setting up interviews with other nursing tutors and a forum for discussion of what I was doing. It was part of my integration back into the nursing establishment.

Not until the end of the first year with a methodology summer school, did the relief and revelation come that other postgraduates had trouble with their filing systems, how to take notes, and how to distinguish fact from opinion in their own writing, let alone other people's. I found that everyone struggled to write, or avoid it, that their theoretical base was not the clear shining light illuminating their path that I assumed it should be. Indeed other participant observers, like me, were at a loss to know how data fits theory or theory fits data. That these were not necessarily difficulties solved as an undergraduate indicated that some of the questions I had thought to be too obvious to ask about were part of learning research. Others too suffered from degrees of lack of professional confidence that I had not formerly thought commensurate with the status of a postgraduate, and as we chatted over the minutiae of our research problems, informally as much as in guided sessions, so our academic contacts grew to good effect and came to be renewed at future conferences. I found this invaluable.

A one-month hospice course during the first year had firmed up my supposition that there was a gap between the rhetoric of 'good' terminal care, and what happens when it is practised, and also indicated some of the future problems of participant observation. As the time for the bulk of the fieldwork was approaching, I anticipated difficulties in writing at the end of a shift. I therefore devised a limited number of A4 forms (to allow for later adaptation) – partly numbers and cases, and partly descriptive, to ease the way into getting the shift into some kind of perspective. To this were to be added tape recordings of what the shift had felt like, although it was only once the fieldwork was underway that sheets of 'odd thoughts' developed. They made no attempt to be a coherent part of the data, but just seemed brilliantly insightful at the time.

Another aspect of preparation was to introduce myself and the study to the hospital ward and the continuing care unit where I was to work – ostensibly to ask their permission, although I felt they had little choice once the doctors and the Ethical Committee had agreed to it.

The sister on the medical ward which was used mainly for heart patients was exceptionally open-minded, forward thinking and relaxed, but saw little point in having a researcher into dying on the ward when there were not that many deaths – which was difficult when the numbers of deaths apparently went up when I was there. The common quip about me being a Jonah had something of an edge to it. In contrast, the sister on the continuing care unit, a place known as something of a deathhouse, was anxious to present the staff and patients as a happy and unified family – which I did not believe, but had qualms at the prospect of exposing. In both places I sat in on the report when all the nurses on duty regularly gather together, to explain what I wanted to do, neither wanting to appear an academic know-all nor to make them feel like the objects of study. (In the end, one of the ways I was accepted was to be thought of as clever (only clever people are at university) but a bit dim at practical things.) I could only explain in general terms what I intended to do, pointing out that the outcome of the research was unclear – it was exactly why I was going to do the study – and so like many researchers, deliberately or not, I failed to convey what the research was about.

To maintain my identity as a researcher, what I wore to work (it was noticeable that I used 'work' to describe nursing but rarely to describe writing or university events) became of symbolic significance. I was in a quandary, as I did not want to deliberately obscure my identity to pretend I was not doing research, but also wanted to be accepted as one of the team, though the administrators wanted me to be visibly different. The white coat was discarded in favour of a nursing dress, but I was not to have a hat or epaulettes which denote the stage and type of training. As was intended these careful omissions generated an awareness of my difference, but by the end of fieldwork in the hospital, before I started in the unit, I had acquired both. Usually reluctant to wear uniforms, not feeling I belonged was disquieting and I made the effort to be allowed the privilege of wearing a white paper hat, and the pink epaulettes of a staff nurse. Going native.

Which is the right information?

The great day came. The proper start of fieldwork. On for an early shift, I got up at 5.30 a.m. after a terrible night's sleep, drove with jumbled thoughts to the hospital, changed in the sisters' locker room (a measure of my confusing status to administrators as well as to myself), and went down early to the ward where my name had been added to the nursing rota. (Despite my being on the rota, no nurse was to be displaced as the result of my being there. It would have caused union problems as I was unpaid. It was also to my advantage because most nurses are reluctant to be 'lent' when there are too many nurses on the ward, and it could have created bad feeling.) The shift was a daunting muddle to me. We had report and unlike the others, I was not allocated to work with someone but left to find my own jobs. The Sister thought she was being helpful, but I felt lost. A few remarks from my fieldnotes:

> I didn't know what I was doing, and the lack of routine was very undermining, or rather the lack of knowledge of the routine was very undermining to me. I felt that I had no independence on the ward because I nearly always had to ask people if I wanted to do, or thought I ought to do, something.

> One of the problems all during today has been the vast input of possible information, and not knowing how to select it. I'd already decided that for the first couple of days I'd concentrate on my own socialization, the acquiring of the routine, learning about the ward and so on to be able to write down the timetable of the nursing day, but even so.

Confusion and doubt is part of any nurse's move to a new ward, but I had forgotten that and I found it difficult to make sense of things as a nurse, let alone a researcher. Even as I settled down to doing auxiliary-nurse-type of work, though still having coffee in Sister's office, I was casting about for what it was that I was trying to discover. Good social scientists manage to establish valuable facts. My observations seemed to lack that authority. And

> ... field researchers always live, to some extent, with the disquieting notion that they are gathering the wrong data, that they should be observing or asking questions about another event or practice, instead of the present one.

Truth, objectivity and bias loomed large in my thinking throughout the fieldwork, and increasingly quantitative research seemed to hold the enticing allure of being 'scientific'. It was not until I was well back out of the nursing that what had been written during it looked as though it had any purpose or explanatory use.

It was intended that the research would generate its own emphases, but I had needed not only a product to sell to the people whose aid I wanted to enlist, but also to give some direction to my thinking – as for instance in the forms I made.

In submitting the proposal to the nursing administrators I had made a mental note to beware that I did not get taken in by my own propaganda, to remember that my interest was skewed to people who were thought to be ill and people who helped look after them, rather than patients and nurses, that I was being a nurse merely as a means to research. Once involved, that seemed heartlessly instrumental. When they went to supper, work stopped for them, as they assumed it did for me, and their trust, which I wanted, was discomforting. Occasionally passing outrageous remarks to make it clear that I was not one of them, giving them a chance to defend themselves against me, did little but salve my conscience. However, as they were subjects of study to me, so to some extent was I subject to study and use by them. In attempting to keep free enough from the restrictions of hypotheses to let the data indicate the important issues, so I was open to be buffeted by the most powerful influences and friendships. The result is that the majority of quotable quotes came from few people, and my preoccupations were those of the places and people with whom I worked. A useful bias . . .

. . .

Unanticipated and useful additions to my knowledge were also made as my status changed, on the hospital ward, but more obviously so in the continuing care unit. In both places I tried to fit in by doing what was asked of me, but not taking leading decisions, and I had thought that I would work in the background with the auxiliaries. Not only do the auxiliaries not stay in the background, but I was known to be a staff nurse. By the fourth day in the hospital, when I asked a student nurse about doing something, she said: 'You decide, you're in charge.' When time was short and the drug round was due, I was qualified to do it, and to take charge of the drug keys when other trained staff were off the ward. Adopting different roles in the hierarchy is what everyone but the most senior do everyday, and that on one shift I could be in charge of the continuing care unit and the next be cleaning the sluice – auxiliary territory – pointed up just how conscious and specific the hierarchies are. . . .

As my time at the hospital came to a close, I decided that a longer and perhaps more reflective discussion on the nurses' thoughts about their work would be a helpful addition to the remarks and brief debates that I heard as they organized and cared for the patients. On night duty there had been more opportunity to talk casually and at length, but on days it needed to be arranged beforehand. I went to Betty's house as researcher and workmate, but after a five-hour rambling conversation which included her husband and child, interspersed with lunch and afternoon tea, the difficulty of remembering what had been said made leaving a tape recorder running an attractive proposition. I asked the Sister if she minded me having one there as she and I talked round a few subjects, and she was relaxed enough to ignore it. I did not do enough taping at the hospital before I left to take account of the kind of effect I was having.

During a two-month break from nursing for a reappraisal of where I'd got so far, I gave a seminar paper in the department which, though not obvious then, became one of the main outlines for the final thesis. This, together with the regular meetings with my supervisor throughout the fieldwork, allowed some of my thoughts on terminal care nursing to coalesce. When I went to work on the purpose-built continuing care unit I hoped, somewhat deviously, that getting people to talk about their thoughts on how care of the dying should be approached would give a helpful comparison with what could be observed of their practice of it. I postponed doing this until I was better known, but when an excellent nurse was about to leave, I was provoked to start. People knew me and my ideas too well for me to be able to interview them, and although there were four general areas I wanted to ask about, having a 'conversation' was more appropriate. Taping saved intrusive scribbling. I anticipated that everyone worked with me and teased me well enough for the conversations not to bother them too much. They were either at people's houses or at the unit, whichever they preferred, but the variations in how easy people found it, and their fluency in the more formal talk, were enormous. Until I listened to the tapes retrospectively, I did not realize the resistance, despite familiarity, of the power structure between interviewer and informant. In some cases I got the power balances quite wrong even when I had learnt to sit through the silences, though in others they organized themselves to make it easier. I arrived at Mary's to find that she had invited Jessica round so they could do it together, and we all had lovely afternoon tea. This in itself was good data, not to be missed out and whilst it was part of the 'gossamer of ideas' on how nurses control their circumstances, I was constantly concerned as to its validity (to whom?) and acceptability (to whom?) as social science, prompted by what I thought to be its unacceptability within medical circles. They obviously talked over the conversations with each other as they happened, and inevitably the discussions gave pause for reflection – I was told so several times – but how they affected behaviour was impossible to detect.

The unit was something of a showcase, built as it was with money from the local community and with the purpose of providing care for cancer patients. The Sister in charge was therefore more involved than most in showing visitors round, thereby, with some anxiety, putting herself on show. She looked after me as thoughtfully as she looked after the others, giving me time in the quiet room to write up notes, and I suspect she was both pleased and somewhat disquieted to have me there. Although we were both careful in our management of it, it is possible that I may have been a threat to her, and as far as I can remember, despite being there for five months, I did not publicly air my views in front of her as vehemently as I did in other chatting groups. Mutual support is an important contribution to maintaining a happy atmosphere in terminal care units, feared and criticized as they often are by outsiders, and stressful within. My criticisms, through regular discussion and deliberate distancing, were more succinct than most, and it was something of a dilemma when asked my opinion.

A dysfunction built into the research, for which I had made inadequate provision, was the constant prodding at the defence mechanisms which are a means of continuing at the unit. If I pushed the others too far they would evade, avoid or tell me to shut up, but my own defences were also under scrutiny and the more I was perturbed by exposing them, the more my reluctance to write up at the end of the day grew. I was enjoying the nursing. For the research, philosophy, the structure of the National Health Service, and numbers became easier lines of thought. None of them had anything to do with people. . . .

## 3

Working with women's health groups: The community health movement

Jean Orr

There is in Britain a growing dynamic and innovatory community health movement. According to Rosenthal (1983) this movement is based outside the health professionals and is concerned with identifying inequalities in health and health care provision. It is based on the belief that the achievement of a healthy community depends on a collective awareness of the social causes of ill health, and it challenges on individual and collective levels the monopoly of information about health and ill health which is controlled by health professionals.

Many of the initiatives in the community health movement concern women. In many communities this trend cuts across class and political groupings and results in the spontaneous *ad hoc* organization of women to meet a particular need or combine against a specific threat. This is evident in the range of self-help and protest groups which have been mushrooming in the past 5–10 years. Examples of these are the Rape Crisis Centres, Women's Aid and Well Women Groups and Centres.

This should come as no surprise to health visitors who must recognize that the matters women most care about, and are responsible for, happen in the home, i.e. in the community (Bayley, 1982). This differs from the world of most men, for whom the core of their life is work and the activities associated with that. Women are very aware that the community they inhabit is not the community idealized by politicians, but it is the place where women are in direct contact and confrontation with the State as represented by housing, welfare and health services. For many women their contact with these services only reinforces their roles and makes implicit and explicit the women's degree of failure. . . .

The fact that women themselves are organizing is indicative of their concern and their determination to bring about change. The women's health movement is a good example of how women have challenged the health care professionals and have spearheaded a nationwide movement. In the north-west of England, for example, there is a strong, articulate body of women who have succeeded in setting up women's health classes and self-help groups and have thus been instrumental in the establishment of well women clinics. While these women are from very diverse backgrounds, they appear united in their demand for health care on their terms.

The well women clinics which have been established are examples of how lay and professional women have changed policies and provided a very different service from that of a cytology or family planning clinic. The emphasis is on helping the women to identify their own health and social needs by taking a holistic approach. Women's health needs, after all, involve more than cervical smears and breast examinations. The women are invited to join a range of self-help groups and attend sessions on specific health problems such as depression.

Women's health groups

Women's health self-help groups are a relatively new aspect of health care in Britain and yet the existence of these groups is a criticism of existing provision. The women's health movement has identified the dissatisfaction which women experience in their interaction with the range of health care services. Many feminist writers express an antagonism to the health care services, which are often seen as a form of social control (Ehrenreich and English, 1973; Daly, 1978).

The growing body of literature on women's health identifies the gap between the professional view of women's health and what is experienced by women in their everyday lives. Much of the literature attempts to redefine women's health and give women control over their bodies and their health (Orr, 1986).

One way women have demonstrated their desire for knowledge is to come together in groups to discuss health issues. It was realized that many women attending the well women clinics had long-term problems and/or had expressed a need to meet together with other women to discuss issues in their lives. Therefore women's health groups developed alongside well women clinics. Many women came long distances to these groups and subsequently campaigned for clinics in their own areas.

Women's health groups also developed in the absence of clinics and in the face of opposition by professional health workers. In one area of Greater Manchester, for example, women were attending well women sessions on health at an average of 150 per night while health visitors were saying there was no need and women would not come to this type of session. Groups were also organized by voluntary and community associations such as the Workers' Education Association.

The women's health movement is made up of a cross-section of women who have demanded and achieved change. We thus have to rethink the stereotypical labelling which suggests that women cannot work together, and that working-class women are inarticulate and passive.

Studying the groups

Over a period of three years I have been involved in working with ten women's health groups in the north-west of England. I came to work with these groups as part of ongoing research into well women clinics and my concern about women's health. This work was, and is, largely an expression of my belief in feminism and from this ensued a commitment to share whatever skills I had with other women. It also became apparent, because of the unique nature of the groups, that there was a need to record and share the group process with other people. In that sense research was an outcome of my involvement, not a reason for it. Nurses and health visitors are in a key position to assist women achieve optimum health, but only if they listen to what women are saying. These groups provided an opportunity to listen to women who were concerned about health but were not likely to make these concerns known to professionals. I was concerned with making these women's experiences visible and influential in affecting changes in health care provision. The only framework which appeared to achieve this was that of feminist research which, according to Webb (1984), changes the nature of the relationship between researcher and researched by making women's experience visible. It does this through the medium of consciousness-raising, asserting that in research as in all social life the personal is the political.

I experienced what Stanley and Wise (1983) discuss when they say that feminist research should be the doing of feminism in another context. The doing of research requires the activities and procedures we use in the ordinary understanding of ourselves as women in the social world.

There is a difficulty in recording the processes of such groups because of the *ad hoc* nature of the membership and the informality of the group. Pre- and post-testing, questionnaires and other structured measurements would have been an intrusion into the group processes and would have deterred participation. For many of these women this experience of the group was intensely personal and as they were self-disclosing aspects of their lives which were often painful much of the group activity was to build trust and create an environment in which these women could feel safe.

I was a participant observer of these groups. The theoretical rationale for the use of participant observation is based on three concepts. Firstly, the basic functionalist perspective of attempting to understand social facts in their wider context encourages the observation of the total life of a community, however defined, rather than the abstraction of selected variables. Secondly, the Weberian tradition in sociology, in stressing the need to define how various social actors in a given context perceive their situation, ascertains that what people believe to be is as significant as that which is, in the understanding of social behaviour. Thirdly, because the phenomena being studied are undergoing continuous change, we need a method for exploring emergent structures. This method could be seen as 'the best fit' for discovery and exploration amidst social change (Glaser and Strauss, 1965).

Therefore the incorporation of the investigator into the social context under study is arguably the best suited to understand how groups perceive, define and react to certain situations. This requires that the researcher should be concerned not only with what is objective, but dialectically with the interrelation of objective and subjective material. This interpretive approach implies that social interaction is to be understood as the construct of processes by which actors and observers make sense out of what is taking place and use this interpretation as grounds for ordering their own actions.

A feminist interviewing women is by definition both inside the culture and participating in that which she is observing, according to Oakley (1981), and so this appeared the best method. When possible I took notes during the group meeting and wrote these up in detail immediately afterwards. I did not want the research to intrude or detract from the group experience. These women were not coming together as a research facility, they were together because of their concerns. It was difficult to see them as 'data'. There is a quality of relations which develop with people involved in a study, and a quality of understanding which emerges from those relations, which is little discussed in traditional (or male) texts or research (Stanley and Wise, 1983). . . .

Description of groups

The groups came into existence in a number of ways, and were very diverse in membership and structure. Three of the groups were set up by the Workers Education Association and ran for six weekly sessions. These were linked to local education schemes and women came to the group while their children were in the play group.

Four groups were set up by the well women's movement, and two of these were linked to well women clinics. Local Community Associations had organized three women's health groups which ran for four weeks.

These groups were unlike anything I had experienced in the National Health Service. Every group was like no other group. Although these are often called self-help groups they were in many ways different. There is no one easy definition of these groups but they seem to be a mixture of consciousness-raising and self-help.

Self-help/consciousness-raising

Consciousness-raising groups are those in which women get together away from men, and work to express and analyse their experience and feelings and to support each other (Radcliffe Richards, 1980). Liberman and Bond (1976) in a study of consciousness-raising groups in the United States, suggest that women attending such groups wanted to share and compare the experience and feelings of women. Consciousness-raising groups are a type of group whose goal is to explore and often seek to change the circumstances of its members. Consciousness-raising groups do not adhere to a centralized structure; they focus on one particular topic for a session and members are encouraged to share their particular experiences. By concentrating on the commonality of women's experience the group encourages members to see that problems are often not caused by personal inadequacy but are based in current social structure. Smith (1980) sees that the potential effect, therefore, is to decrease self-blame for past and present failings and to offer support to members in changing aspects of their lives. The pooling of experience should reduce the degree of isolation felt by many women, and should help them to feel confident in asserting their needs to others (Ernst and Goodison, 1981).

There is an emphasis in consciousness-raising groups that everyone's feelings are of equal importance. It is, according to Radcliffe Richards (1980), a most important insight of feminism to realize that the least articulate women are very likely to be the most oppressed. Difficulty in self-expression is taken to mean that a woman has nothing worth saying.

Some women's health groups lay emphasis on teaching self-help skills such as breast or pelvic examination and the use of alternative therapies such as massage. The group I was involved with did not, but this may develop as it has done in other parts of Britain and America. The groups shared many of the characteristics of self-help and consciousness-raising groups, although the women who attended were in no sense radical. Smith (1980) says that the effectiveness of self-help groups and consciousness-raising groups has been little studied but it probably rests upon the experience of continual support. In the case of the women's groups effectiveness can be seen in this light. It could also be argued that the activity of group members to campaign for more groups or well women clinics is a measure of success.

The groups were organized and operated outside the health care facilities and although in the north-west health workers were involved, they had no special status.

My role was to lead these groups, so in that sense they were not truly self-help. But the aim was to start off the discussion and encourage maximum participation by the members and give them the opportunity to share feelings and validate experiences.

The topics advertised in the programmes included, diet, depression, premenstrual tension, menopause, cystitis, motherhood, contraception, exercise and relaxation. Posters were displayed in clinics, libraries, community centres, and shopping centres.

Findings

Some women came for all sessions; others attended once or twice. Numbers varied considerably. One meeting on depression was attended by 150 women, one on diet by 30. The usual membership was between seven and ten. This wide range of membership made it necessary to adapt the sessions. It is not possible to have the same level of discussion in a room of 150 women as it is in a small group of eight. Most importantly the content of the discussion often bore very little relationship to the advertised topic. Unlike, for example, ante-natal classes which are 'teacher-led' these sessions were structured to explore issues of importance to the women. The group proceeded at its own pace and the content matched the women's needs. Therefore a session on contraception developed into a discussion of female sexuality and sexual difficulties. A session on mothering developed into a discussion on women's role within the family and the experience of being the victim of violence. This was the first time the majority of these women had had the opportunity to discuss such issues, and to recognize that their personal experience was shared by others. As one woman said, 'I didn't know other women felt like me about sex – he told me I was frigid and no good.' Another said, 'When you're shut away in your own house there's no-one to talk to – I felt I was going crazy because I couldn't stand my kids all day and I thought it was just me.'

This process of consciousness-raising was very painful, although the women involved may not have come to a group which was labelled anything other than health.

The 'health topic' legitimized the women's attendance. For these women it was only permissible to go out if they were going to be 'improved', e.g. have their premenstrual tension reduced, and be easier to live with. This points up two features of these women's lives, which were discussed in the groups. Firstly there are very few places for these women to go and meet other women in a safe environment, and secondly such outings as are possible have to be seen as self-improving for the benefit of the family which in many cases means the male partner.

Case studies of two groups

Group A

Group A met in a church hall in a very deprived part of Manchester. A local community education scheme organized the group in conjunction with the local play group. There were eight young women attending from the local estate; all had one child, four were single mothers and all were dependent on benefits. The topic which was to be discussed was 'How to be a mother and stay sane'. This was the first time I had met these women and I introduced myself as being interested in women's health.

The most disconcerting feature of this group of women was that they did not act as it is assumed groups should act. They got up and walked about, talked to each other and generally ignored me. They had never been in a group before and had not 'learnt' the rules. The rules therefore had to change rapidly. I started to talk to two women who were sitting together, and after 15 minutes other women began to join us. Women moved in and out of this small group and pursued conversations of their own. It was near the end of the 1½-hour session before we all came together and formed what most textbooks would call 'a group'.

While these women had experiences of health services through having children, they had little belief that these services were of any benefit to them or were in any sense relevant to their concerns. All of the women talked of being severely depressed after the birth of their children, and none had received help from their doctors. Two had obviously been identified as at-risk because the health visitor called weekly. 'She calls every week – she's nice and young and I can talk to her – but you don't tell her about this – they'd take the baby away.'

Indeed the women were right because the stories they told of trying to kill their babies would have resulted in action by the statutory services.

> I got piano wire and took it in to the Prem nursery to cut off its head – I was never alone with him but every day I wanted to do it. I didn't want him home.

> I left it out in the rain to drown it and put her in the coal shed one night she wouldn't stop crying.

> I wanted to iron my little girl's face – she wouldn't stop crying – my mother caught me with the iron and sat on me for a couple of days until I was better. I'd like another kid but I couldn't go through that horrible depression again. I know I was crazy.

Because these women had known each other for some time they joined in and reinforced each other's experience by telling of mutual help and support. Family and friends had been the only acceptable help for these women. They would not consider statutory services could help them because of their distrust of State intervention and past experiences with the services. For these women the only source of help which would be acceptable would be in an informal setting with women from their own area.

These women did not attend ante-natal or child health clinics. They saw no point in it and felt ill at ease in those settings. They did, however, want to do their best for their children and were interested in their own health. For them the idea of someone as the expert made them feel inadequate.

Stanley and Wise (1983) reject the idea that we can become experts in other people's lives and reject the belief that there is one true real reality to become experts about. It may be that these women will only accept help in this type of setting and the role of professional may be to facilitate these types of groups by providing information and working with lay women.

There are problems in professionals being involved in self-help groups, because the group members' experience may have led to a distrust of authoritarian nature of professional activity (Borman, 1976). No matter how much the professional wishes to step out of this mould the client's perceptions may be such that this is impossible.

There is little evidence that existing types of ante-natal or post-natal groups would appeal to these women, and perhaps we have to recognize that for some women help needs to be offered through this type of informal group organized outside the health services.

Group B

This was a group of women between 45 and 60 years old and three women of about 20, who were attending a 2-hour session on the menopause. This session formed part of a series on general health issues organized by the Workers' Education Association. The older women were reticent to talk at first, and said they had very little experience of groups. The younger women said they came because they were interested in the menopause and wanted to learn more about it for themselves and their mothers and friends. These women were dressed in punk clothes and contrasted with the older women's more conservative appearance. The older women appeared suspicious and ill at ease with these younger women. Within health care women only come together in specific age ranges, e.g. ante-natal classes, and there is not much opportunity outside the family for cross-generational exchange of what it means to be women in our society.

The younger women had experienced sharing thoughts and feelings in other group settings; the older women had not.

As leader I shared with the group some of my own personal experiences which were relevant and this self-disclosure appeared to give them permission to speak.

This older group of women, like the women in group A, had little contact with health services other than general practice, and this did not meet their needs.

My doctor never listens – he says it's what I can expect at my age.

You don't bother your doctor; he isn't interested in women's complaints.

I came because I'm desperate to talk to someone about whether I should have a hysterectomy or not.

The group was seen as a way of getting information, and as somewhere to get counselling help with specific problems. The group therefore acted as an entry for these women into the women's health services or health advice agencies.

When I saw the title I thought that's for me – they'll know what to do about the hot sweats and all.

But there were other issues which came out of the discussion not specifically related to the menopause. For example a woman who had been a ward sister and was married to a psychologist told us about her concerns – concerns which she had been unable to tell her doctor who was treating her for depression.

My husband made me feel I was crazy because I couldn't cope with money – he wanted a choice of meals every night and I knew if I didn't please him I'd get . . . well he's got a terrible temper. He treats me like a doormat and my two sons are doing the same. I've made my decision to stay with him, what else can I do? My doctor doesn't understand – there's nowhere else to go.

Within our health service there are few outlets for a woman with these problems. She did not feel it was appropriate to attend a family planning or cytology clinic as she had had a hysterectomy.

This woman was referred to a counsellor at one of the well women clinics. The older women talked about a great sense of loss following both hysterectomy and menopause. Scarf (1980) argues that women at 'pressure points' in their lives such as menopause are faced with the task of being alone and having to overcome feelings of separation and loss. For many this can bring to the surface previous unresolved separation crises, and this unfinished business can result in depression. For these women to recognize the unfinished business may help them to overcome depression. It was obviously very painful for many of them and three of the women started to cry. The other group members comforted them.

To give these women the opportunity to express their grief was an important function of the group, but it also highlighted the need to offer continued support in some form. The women agreed to meet outside of the group and to attend a well women clinic. Like the women in group A these women would have wanted information and help, but existing services did not seem to have been appropriate or available. Many of their concerns arose from misleading or incomplete information from medical and nursing staff in hospital.

Conclusion

Throughout the groups there were common features: members had only marginal involvement with health services and had experienced severe problems related to health/social aspects of their lives. They were anxious for help with these aspects of their lives but preferred more informal, less hierarchical structure. They wanted to come together with women who shared their experiences and who took their concerns seriously. Health visitors have to be aware of the literature which should inform practice.

There is a growing body of feminist literature which has relevance to health visiting. This literature identifies women's issues in relation to health care and may have implications for clients' expectations and the way they use health services.

Kjervik and Martinson (1979) bring together work which offers a nursing perspective for women in stress, and suggest that women in nursing should grasp, both personally and professionally, the health care issues confronting women. As women themselves, nurses have added insight into the stress and concerns facing a female client. With their knowledge and self-awareness they can help ease the tension facing women; tensions inherent in divorce, role expectations, battering, child abuse and the stress of loss.

Studies of women's needs have traditionally centred on motherhood, but now include issues which are much broader and affect many aspects of women's lives. Examples of feminist writings include coping with sexual identity crises after mastectomy (Kent, 1975), the need for education in sexuality for nursing (Krizinofski, 1973), the effect of feminism on psychiatry (Coppolillo, 1975) and the grieving process of battered women (Weingourt, 1979).

The relationship between health visiting and women's health will remain tenuous and uneasy unless health visitors make use of this increasing body of literature. Feminism has provided concepts about women's roles and women's health which are crucial to health visitor education and practice, and which helps us to understand and analyse everyday situations.

There is a role for health visitors to be involved in such groups (Drennen, 1985) but the level of that involvement will have to vary according to the group needs, and in certain circumstances may be one of facilitation rather than participation.

References

Bayley, M. (1982). 'Community care and the elderly', in *Care in the Community* (ed. F. Glendenning). Department of Adult Education, University of Keele.

Borman, L. (1976). Self help and the professional. *Social Policy*, 7, 46–47.

Coppolillo, H. (1975). The feminist movement; implications for psychiatry and the family. *Journal of the Tennessee Medical Association*, 68(7), 536–540.

Daly, M. (1978). *Gynecology. The Metaethics of Radical Feminism.* Beacon Press, Boston.

Du Bois, B. (1983). 'Passionate scholarship: notes on values, knowing and method in feminist social science', in *Theories of Women's Studies* (eds G. Bowles and R. Duelli Klein). Routledge & Kegan Paul, London.

Duelli Klein, R. (1983). 'How to do what and we want to do; thoughts about feminist methodology', in *Theories of Women's Studies* (eds G. Bowles and R. Duelli Klein). Routledge & Kegan Paul, London.

Ehrenreich, B. and English, D. (1973). *Complaints and Disorders: the sexual politics of sickness.* Feminist Press, New York.

Ernst, S. and Goodison, L. (1981). *In Our Own Hands: a book of self help therapy.* Women's Press, London.

Evans, M. (1983). 'In praise of theory; the case for women's studies', in *Theories of Women's Studies* (eds G. Bowles and R. Duelli Klein). Routledge & Kegan Paul, London.

Glaser, B. and Strauss, A. (1965). 'Discovery of substantive theory: a basic strategy underlying qualitative research', in *Qualitative Methodology* (ed. W. Filstead). Markham, Chicago.

Kent, S. (1975). Coping with sexual identity crises after mastectomy. *Geriatrics*, 30(10), 145–146.

Kjervik, D. and Martinson, J. (1979). *Women in Stress: a nursing perspective.* Appleton-Century-Crofts, New York.

Krizinofski, M. (1973). Human sexuality and nursing practice. *Nursing Clinics of North America*, 8(4), 673–681.

Liberman, M. and Bond, G. (1976). The problem of being a woman. *Journal of Applied Behavioural Science*, 12, 363–379.

Orr, J. (ed.) (1986). *Women's Health in the Community.* John Wiley & Sons, London.

Radcliffe Richards, N. (1980). *The Sceptical Feminist.* Penguin, Harmondsworth.

Rosenthal, H. (1983). Neighbourhood health projects. Some new approaches to health and community work in parts of the United Kingdom. *Community Developmental Journal*, 18(2), 120–131.

Scarf, M. (1980). *Unfinished Business*. Fontana, Glasgow.

Smith, P. (1980). *Group Processes and Personal Change*. Harper & Row, London.

Stanley, L. and Wise, S. (1979). Feminist research, feminist consciousness and experience of sexism. *Women's Studies International Quarterly*, 2(3), 359–379.

Stanley, L. and Wise, S. (1983). 'Back into the personal or our attempt to construct feminist research', in *Theories of Women's Studies* (eds G. Bowles and R. Duelli Klein). Routledge & Kegan Paul, London.

Webb, C. (1984). Feminist methodology in nursing research. *Journal of Advanced Nursing*, 9(3), 248–256.

Weingourt, R. (1979). Battered women and the grieving process. *Journal of Psychiatric Nursing*, 17(4), 40–47.

☰ Section B ☰

Talking to people and asking questions

Introduction

The four chapters in this section are about gathering data by asking people questions, as opposed to working with them and seeing how things are done – participant observation – as illustrated in Section A. The chapters differ along a continuum of structure. In the first, very little preconception is imposed on the topic, and the method of interviewing is generally described as *open* or *ethnographic*. Women are asked about their lives and experiences and encouraged to talk about themselves and their histories in their own terms; there is a research agenda, but the researchers make every effort not to let it alter what the informants want to say about themselves. (A fair amount of this kind of interviewing, and less formal 'chats', goes on in participant observation research as well, as you will have realized from Kirkham's and James' chapters in Section A.)

The crucial stage of research is the beginning, when the important decisions are taken which will affect what can be concluded from our work. Chapter 5 in this section describes the planning stage of a piece of research into heart patients from a District General Hospital in the South of England and the consequences of the trip to London some of them have to make for treatment; the research aims to provide understanding of how much this trip disrupts their and their families' lives and to gather information which can be used to improve services to such patients. It outlines some of the decisions that had to be made and some of the alternative approaches which had to be discarded. It demonstrates how sampling is worked out in a real-life situation and how groups are selected for comparison, to maximize the 'pay-off' from the data. It also raises some of the ethical issues which researchers face at the design stage.

Chapter 6 describes a formal survey in which categories of 'user' of a hospital (including the staff) are asked predetermined direct questions about their experience of open visiting and its problems. The idea of a survey is that all the respondents are asked the same structured questions in the same way – presented with a constant stimulus – so that differences between their answers are due to differences in their character or experience, not differences in the way the information was collected. (We talk about surveys as ways of asking structured *questions*, but the same principles hold for surveys in which the researcher systematically *observes* what is going on in, e.g. different school playgrounds or different magistrates' courts or different casualty departments; survey data do not have to be verbal.) Chapter 7, an attitude study, uses a still more highly structured form of data-collection, the Semantic Differential, as a way of eliciting attitude material without directly asking attitudinal questions – deducing attitudes from scores on a measuring instrument which is deliberately made vague and ambiguous from the informant's point of view.

The strengths of Chapters 6 and 7 – and of structured surveys in general – are that we have precisely comparable data for all informants, neatly categorized to facilitate comparison. Their weakness is that the data are categorized in terms of the researchers' conception of the topic area, which is not necessarily the same as the informants'. This makes them good tools for testing researchers' hypotheses that specified groups will answer preset questions in predictably different ways – to test theory, in other words – but not necessarily very apt for exploration and theory-*building*. The open interviewing technique used in Chapter 4 is better adapted to exploring how the informants see their worlds in their own terms, but the price paid for this richness of data is that it may be more difficult to compare across cases.

The difference between Chapter 4 and these two reflects a traditional divide in discussions about research methods – between 'qualitative' and 'quantitative' work. The former, exemplified by Abbott and Sapsford in Chapter 4, owes a primary commitment to naturalism and holism. That is, it aims to be able to generalize directly from the research situation to the informants' everyday lives by imposing as little structure as possible on the situation and concentrating in the first instance in letting the informants' own voices be heard. The latter, exemplified by Chapters 6 and 7, owes a primary commitment to reliable and generalizable description and/or the testing of hypotheses. The difference in *naturalism* is one of degree, not of kind, in these chapters. The chapter on hospital visiting (Chapter 6), for instance, tries to ask its questions in language which is natural for the informants, as if a naturalistic conversation were taking place. On the other hand, open interviewing is not unstructured, any more than any conversation is unstructured. Indeed, detailed analysis of open interviews reveals a degree of structure which would not be natural for an everyday conversation, with the researcher contributing far less information to the conversation than would be normal but taking far greater charge of it in the sense of determining when the subject is to be changed and when a topic needs further elaboration. The difference in *holism* is perhaps more than a matter of degree, however: the 'open interviewing' chapter (Chapter 4) tries to set the research topic in the context of the whole lives of the participants, while the other two have predetermined areas of enquiry with which they are designed to deal in predetermined ways and using predetermined questions exploring *aspects* which are thought to be relevant.

Differences in approach are to some extent independent of method, however, as is demonstrated by the way the different papers approach the cluster of attitudes/beliefs/opinions. How you measure or collect these depends on how you conceptualize them. If you think of an attitude or a belief as something 'factual' – something the person has, is aware of and can report – then the simplest thing is to ask direct questions as in Chapter 6: 'Have you ever been bothered by other people's visitors?'. Alternatively, however, you could undertake open interviewing from this stance, with the same intention of taking what people said about their lives as a factual and authoritative report, true because they say it is true. If you think of attitudes as something which people have but of which they are not necessarily aware – implicit ways of judging the world or tendencies to behave in certain ways – then you might use a more indirect method such as the semantic differential scales of Chapter 7, trying to uncover what lies *underneath* the explicit judgements that people make. Alternatively, you might undertake open interviewing, but with the intention of interpreting what was said rather than taking it at face value. If you believe that attitudes are something that people *do* – ways in which they make sense to themselves of their actions and their experiences – then you would be most likely to undertake open interviewing, to see how they form and express opinions in context-specific ways. You might, however, use either of the other approaches, but be inclined to interpret the results more cautiously and reflexively than if you held one of the other positions.

In one respect, then, these chapters differ in the degree of structure which they exhibit. In another, however, they are all fairly structured; the nature of the informants is carefully managed to suit the 'argument' of the research. Chapter 5 is entirely about how a piece of research was structured in practice, as a compromise between the ideal and the practical. Chapter 6, on hospital visiting, sets out to cover all interested parties – patients, visitors, nurses – and so the informants are selected to fall into and be representative of these groups. It also has a comparison group – the gynaecological wards, whose clients are similar to those on maternity – to show whether what is experienced on the maternity wards is specific to them or common to other settings. Chapter 7, on attitudes of male and female nurses, has a natural structure built into its subject matter: it compares males with females. The first, though the most qualitative of the papers, has the greatest degree of structuring in terms of its samples. Being concerned with the experiences of mothers of children with learning difficulties, the researchers naturally seek out a sample of such mothers. Being aware, however, that you cannot say what is specific to such mothers unless you can show differences from other kinds of mother, the researchers make an effort to find a group of mothers whose children are not labelled in this way, to act as a comparison. Although we think of qualitative research as unstructured, this kind of theoretical sampling to explore the extent to which the results are correctly understood is entirely typical both of open interviewing research and of participant observation. Comparison and contrast lie at the centre of our understanding of data; we do not understand our results until we know precisely to whom they do or do not apply.

Again, one would traditionally expect survey work to exhibit a fair amount of care over demonstrating that samples are typical of the population which they purport to represent. (It is a fault of Choon and Skevington in Chapter 7 that they do not do so; we are not told how the male and female nurses are selected and therefore cannot judge how typical they were of male and female nurses in general.) Broadly speaking, there are five methods of assuring representation in the selection of respondents.

1. The easiest way is, of course, not to sample at all but to try to approach everyone, as in a census, and this is the approach taken by Abbott and Payne (Chapter 6) when approaching hospital staff – the questionnaire was sent to every member of staff in the maternity and gynaecology units.
2. Given that sampling is necessary, the best method is *random sampling*, where a list of the population is prepared and cases are chosen from it randomly until the desired size of sample is obtained. There can be no conscious bias in such sampling, because the researcher does not control who is chosen. If the sample is reasonably large there should also be little accidental bias, because the likelihood of drawing from one extreme by chance should be balanced by the likelihood of drawing from the opposite extreme.
3. If random sampling is not possible, perhaps because it is not possible to list the entire population, then different methods must be used. In Chapter 6 by Abbott and Payne, where the task was to sample patients and visitors, the researchers originally tried for all visitors and patients present during a certain delimited time period, but had in the end to settle for sampling time periods until enough responses had been obtained. They had therefore to pay some attention to obtaining a spread of time periods, so as not to miss people who visited in the evenings or at weekends. Under other circumstances we might sample an unknown population by taking geographical clusters (streets, houses, post codes) and using these as the contact points for our sample. Again we would have to ensure that we had a good spread of contact points and were not, for example, biased towards middle-class or working-class areas. Properly done, this kind of sampling can produce something which imitates a random sampling method quite well, but inevitably with a slightly higher chance of obtaining a biased (unrepresentative) sample.
4. Where even this is not possible, perhaps for reasons of cost, researchers will sometimes set up what is known as a *quota sample* design. Here you pick important variables whose population distribution is known (e.g. gender, age, class), work out how may people there ought to be in each 'cell' of the design if the sample is to resemble the population (e.g. how many young middle-class males, young middle-class females, middle-aged middle-class males, etc.) and send interviewers out to obtain that number of responses, setting no other constraint on how they find the respondents. This method is widely used in market research and also in political opinion research, where it is said to work quite well. You can imagine, however, that it is

open to introducing very great biases, because interviewers are free to go for
the respondents who are easiest to find at the time when they are looking,
and these may not be typical of the population as a whole.
5. The worst sampling design of all is exhibited by studies which just stop
people in the street, or go from house to house on a particular day, or use
some group who just happen to be available (e.g. a class of students). It is
overwhelmingly likely that these will not form a representative sample.

A final question to consider when evaluating these chapters, therefore, is
whether the samples are representative, and what they represent. Chapter 5 is
reasonably sound in this respect, providing the intended sample can be
achieved. Chapter 6 sets out to represent patients, visitors and staff in the
maternity and gynaecology wards of a major hopsital, and the research is so
structured that it succeeds fairly well in representing visitors and patients. (We
should note, however, that the patients are in part selected by nurses, which
introduces potential biases). It is less successful in representing staff, because
they were left to fill in the questionnaire themselves and return it to the
researchers, and disappointingly few did so. (This would not matter if those
who responded were typical of the remainder, but we have no good reason to
assert unequivocally that this is the case. It is a very common problem of postal
and other 'self-completion' surveys, where response rates of less than 50 per
cent are not at all uncommon.) More broadly, the application of the results
beyond the particular hospital rests on our acceptance that the hospital is
typical of others – not an unreasonable proposition, but one which might
need to be explored before one translated the local results into national policy.
Chapter 7 might be considered as a survey of male and female nurses, but if so
then it lacks the attention to sampling that we would normally expect of
surveys: the males and females sampled are those who happened to be available, with little thought as to whether they are typical. Chapter 4 tries to find a
typical group in the sense that every effort is made to cover a range of 'types'
and circumstances, but there is no good reason to suppose that these few informants constitute a group which reflects exactly the social and personal characteristics of the population of mothers of children with learning difficulties. It is
a good sample for generating description and theory, but to determine relative
frequencies of characteristics in the population a different kind of research
would be needed.

## 4

Leaving it to mum: 'Community care' for mentally handicapped children

Pamela Abbott and Roger Sapsford

The policy of 'community care' for mentally handicapped children has non-financial costs for families: work which in institutions would be wage-labour becomes unpaid work for 'Mum' when the burden of care is transferred to the family. This paper looks at the nature and extent of such work and at the extent to which it alters the nature of the mother's life. We look also at the price which is paid by the whole family for the fact of having a mentally handicapped member – a price made up of shattered expectations which have to be rebuilt, the disturbance to family life, the reactions of others, the constraints on the mother's life, and the disturbance of normal expectations for the family's future. (The 'price' differs markedly from family to family, depending at least in part on the degree of handicap, the extent of associated physical handicaps and the social and economic situation of the family; what follows is a composite, not necessarily true to the experience of any one mother.)

The data come from two main sources. One is research which we carried out jointly during 1981 and 1982 in and around a new city in the English midlands, interviewing mothers of mentally handicapped children (and sometimes other family members who happened to be present). Sixteen families were contacted from a list extracted for us from the school rolls of two Special Schools in the new city (one designated for the mildly handicapped and one for the severely). We carried out two interviews with each mother separated by about a year, not using a formal questionnaire but rather trying for the atmosphere of a friendly chat about life and work between neighbours. Although the interviews were tape-recorded, it seemed to us that this atmosphere was readily attained in most cases – the more so because Abbott was very evidently pregnant during the early interviews. This was one main source of our information. The other source was a similar series of interviews carried out earlier by Abbott with families in an outer London suburb, contacted through

the good offices of the local branch of the National Society for Mental Handicap. Although we cannot claim that either of these small-scale studies has a
sample statistically representative of the population of mentally handicapped
children, we would claim that together they cover a large part of the range –
from the mildest of borderline handicaps to the very severe, and from pre-
school children to (in Abbott's study) 'children' in their forties. These data are
contrasted with a parallel series of interviews with mothers of children who
have *not* been labelled as mentally handicapped.

Reactions to handicap

One major set of costs to the family of the mentally handicapped child is the
reactions which the family will have and will encounter to the fact that their
child is handicapped. The family has to come to terms with altered expectations for the child, an altered perspective for the future, and the cultural stigma
which attaches to the label. A family 'lifestyle' has to be built which can cope
with the situation – and revised, and re-revised as time goes on. Finally, the
family has to negotiate its position *vis-à-vis* the outside world and to deal with
the real, expected or imagined reations of others. This section looks at the
price the family pays for its 'abnormal' member and at how family members
cope with it.

The initial reaction may vary from grief to outright emotional rejection. On
the one hand grief may be immediate and temporarily overwhelming:

> [The Doctor] was rather brutal. I mean true enough one has to learn . . .
> but I left that surgery in tears . . . and I walked and I was crying as I
> walked along.
>
> (Mrs Neade)

Grief may be delayed but no less powerful when it does come: two of the sixteen mothers to whom we spoke described long periods (in one case two or
three years) of numbness, followed by some kind of breakdown. For others
again there may be a period during which the child is effectively rejected:

> For about a month after I found out I didn't have any feeling for her any
> way – she wasn't my baby, she was just *a* baby that had got to be looked
> after and fed and kept clean. I couldn't pick her up and cuddle her or
> nothing . . . And I walked past the pram one day and she looked up at me
> and she smiled at me . . . she just smiled . . . after that I was all right.
>
> (Mrs Miller)

Immediate expectations are broken, and there may be disappointment and
jealously:

> Four girls, five girls who I went to school with . . . all had beautiful
> bouncing babies, and there was me with my poor little thing. I was a bit
> resentful.
>
> (Mrs Miller)

I was most disappointed, because I thought I was going to have a beauti-
ful-looking baby, you know. Well, she was all colours, she was bleeding
all over.

(Mrs King)

Immediate decisions have to be taken: to take the child home or to leave 'it' in
the hospital, to seek or not to seek institutionalization after the child has
gone home, to take all the small decisions which may appear to happen
automatically – 'It's just part of something that happens and you just get on
with it . . . you don't think about each day, do you?' – but which amount to a
commitment to care in the community. The beginnings of a stance towards the
outside world have also to be adopted: for example, the decision not to attempt
concealment:

the sooner people knew, I thought, the nicer for them, because there's
nothing worse than looking in a pram and it's a friend, and thinking, 'Oh
goodness, what can I say'

(Mrs Rushden)

Thus the first thing that has to be done by the family is to come to terms with
broken expectations and altered circumstances – to do the hard work of
building the beginnings of the new and different life. At this time there may
also have to be a reassessment of self. Whether or not the feeling is judged
irrational, there may be a denigration of self – 'I felt inadequate, I felt it must
be me' (Mrs Miller) – and a need to construct some answer to the question
'Why me?'. Seven of our sixteen mothers mentioned some kind of 'hereditary
taint' as something for which one or the other side of the family needed to take
some blame – a survival in popular consciousness of the outdated science of
the Eugenics Movement – and three others denied a belief in heredity with
enough vehemence that one suspects the question had been an issue for the
family. Fathers also may have to come to terms with 'being the sort of person'
who has produced a mentally handicapped child – self-labelling can run all
the more rampant because this is an area of life where it is difficult for spouses
even to talk to each other, let alone talk to others outside the family – and
siblings may worry about themselves and have their worries reinforced by
their school friends.

All of the mothers in our new city sample had made some kind of initial
working adjustment, but the same was not true of all of their husbands. Three
of the sixteen marriages broke up after the birth of the handicapped child –
not solely because of the child's handicap, but at least in part because the
husband could not accept it – and in another case the marriage was put under
great strain. Most of the husbands of the women we have interviewed are
described by their wives as having difficulty in coming to terms with themselves and their children, and in general it is found that stress similar in degree
to the mothers but different in kind (less self-punitive, on the whole) may be
detected in most fathers of mentally handicapped children (Cummings,
1976). Husbands sometimes have to change their lifestyle radically in order to

facilitate the adjustment of the family. Sometimes the husband's job or career has to be modified: for example, one man in our new city sample gave up several chances of promotion to save moving to another area, and another took on a fish and chip shop, with his wife, in order to be more available to the family. Substantial reorganization of normally expected roles may be necessary to preserve an otherwise normal family life: siblings may have to take on a parental role with respect to the handicapped child, and the husband may have to play more of a part in family life than is the norm.

The literature suggests that on the whole fathers become more involved in child care than those whose children are not mentally handicapped. In a survey carried out by Hunter (1980), for example, 25 per cent of employed fathers of mentally handicapped children were 'on nights' or on shift work, and therefore available to take children to clinics and in general to look after them during the day; some fathers had changed to shift work precisely for this reason. On the other hand, some studies find the opposite: Gallagher *et al.* (1983), for example, note that 'the father often plays a limited role in these families even when present'. Both in our new city sample and in the earlier South London work the predominant experience was nearer to the latter state than the former – fathers did help with children, but in general no more so than might be found in some other families. The immediate stress of handicap is in any case less for employed fathers than for non-working mothers because they escape from home for substantial periods of the day. The relationship between husband and wife may well deteriorate nonetheless, as we have seen.

Thus one major 'price' which the parents of mentally handicapped children have to pay for their children is a reorganization of how the family sees itself and how life is lived within it and in interaction with others around it. A second, related price is paid in terms of the nature of the family's identity *vis-à-vis* the outside world and the consequent reactions of others. Mental handicap is a stigmatizing condition in our culture, and it is not only the retarded themselves who carry the stigma, but also their families. Goffman (1963) refers to the sharing of another's spoilt identity as 'bearing a courtesy stigma' – the family members have a spoilt identity because of their close affiliation to someone who bears the primary signs. Birenbaum (1970) suggests that the families of the mentally subnormal tend to provide a very good example of a group of people who carry this kind of courtesy stigma but who seek to maintain a normal appearance by carrying on with the 'normal' life pattern. In order to do this they maintain a 'normal' family life, avoid stigmatizing situations and retain social relationships. Sometimes this may mean a dramatic change in the nature of the social relations which are retained. The South London sample, for instance, were all active members of their local association and tended to use it as a basis for the family's social life. This was much less common among our later new city sample – the local association was far less active there – but many of the mothers at least were actively involved with the teachers and social workers of the ESN(S) school or with the newly formed parents' association at the ESN(M) school. Several mothers were also active in charitable work for the mentally handicapped – Mrs Neade, for example, had until recently been a local organizer for Home Farm Trust's fund-raising activities, and Mrs Rushden was involved in so many things that she described mental handicap as her hobby. While some were well integrated in villages or urban communities, and others in a state of 'normal' urban isolation, others tended to shape their friendships around their retarded children. In Mrs Ovenden's words,

> I miss my friends. Nearly all my friends now are mothers who have children with difficulties, from the [ESN(M)] school, and they've been a great help. But some of the others! One woman kept trying to put Clive down by getting her own child (the same age) to show him how to do things. He doesn't worry, of course, but I mind . . .

In any case the problem of integration tends to become greater as the child reaches adulthood and it becomes increasingly difficult to retain an appearance of normality.

The experiences of the eleven families interviewed in the South London study varied considerably. Some felt intensely that they were stigmatized as a consequence of having a handicapped member and that other people openly displayed negative reactions towards them. These negative reactions might be displayed by relatives, friends, the 'general public' and professionals alike. Conversely others felt that everyone had been very helpful and kind. Abbott's own impressions – from looks, inflections in the voice and other cues as well as from what people said – were that they had all had disturbing experiences and that they all felt that other people regarded them as 'different', pitied them and to some extent avoided them. Also they all seemed to structure their lives as families so as to avoid possibly embarrassing situations – for example, by not asking friends to babysit, by not inviting friends or relatives to call who they felt would be embarrassed by the presence of the subnormal member. What came over most clearly was a feeling that people's attitudes were ambivalent: that at an abstract level they experienced sympathy but that when confronted with the possibility of direct contact with the mentally handicapped they tried to avoid it. Out new city data would admit of a similar analysis.

One has to remember that the majority of people have no first-hand knowledge of the mentally handicapped. They have stereotyped images, often influenced by outdated 'scientific' knowledge and occasionally stirred up by sensationalized newspaper articles. (Attitudes towards sex and the mentally handicapped, discussed below, are a good example of this tendency.) These images more often refer to the severely than to the mildly subnormal. Shearer (1972), for example, has suggested that

> it is still widely believed that mentally handicapped people are uncontrolled and perverted in their sexual appetites. In the past this belief has been one of the main incentives for shutting them away in segregated institutions.

(p. 3)

and Greengross (1976) that

> the fearful myth that the mentally sick and subnormal . . . are promis-
> cuous and have voracious sexual appetites which they are incapable of
> satisfying responsibly or within a socially acceptable pattern of behav-
> iour is one that still holds water for many, and although statistics keep
> pouring out to explode the myth, old prejudices and fears die hard.
>
> (p. 94)

This would seem to be a good example of how arguments developed by the
Eugenics Movement and others to justify the permanent segregation of mentally handicapped people have filtered through and still influence people's
perceptions of the mentally handicapped. The 'outdated' views referred to in
the above quotations were clearly expressed in books and articles on the
mentally subnormal in the first two decades of this century. However, the
view that at least some mentally subnormal men and women have abnormal
appetites is still openly stated by 'experts'. Tredgold and Soddy's influential
textbook for the medical profession argued as recently as 1970 that in the case
of subnormal men

> open masturbation in the presence of others, indecent exposure, inde-
> cent assault especially on immature girls, occasional rape and sexual
> murder are possible.
>
> (p. 90)

while in the case of

> subnormal girls . . . in some ways the problems . . . are even more
> intractable. . . . Some subnormal girls have comparatively strong direct
> sex drives. . . . The gratification aspects of their sexuality will be upper-
> most. Some girls will discover how to use their bodies to give them power
> over men and drift into prostitution. . . . The self-gratification aspects of
> their need can also drive girls into sexual promiscuity.
>
> (p. 91)

(There is indeed some evidence that mentally handicapped men commit more
than their fair share of sexual offences, and that although they are not very
often violent their victims are often young children. However, the total numbers of mentally handicapped men charged and convicted of such offences are
very small – see Walker and McCabe, 1973.)

While scientific and social developments in the twentieth century have
resulted in changes in the way the mentally handicapped are conceptualized
and in methods of handling, nonetheless the beliefs of the Eugenics Movement
live on to a large extent in 'popular consciousness'. The prevalence and power
of the stereotype is well illustrated by a study described by one of us (Abbott,
1982) of a village's reactions to the establishment of a hostel for mentally
handicapped women. While many of the villagers objected vociferously to the
hostel and expressed fears for the safety of the village's children, what was
most revealing was the ambivalent attitudes of a group who became 'Friends

of the Hostel' and visited the girls regularly. Even these women had doubts about whether the hostel should have been opened in their village and in fact shared many of the fears that they claimed were voiced by those opposed to the hostel – fears of violent and sexually uncontrolled behaviour. Similar attitudes and prejudices emerged in group dicussions which Abbott ran with full-time students in a college of further education, a generation on from the 'Friends of the Hostel' and a group selected as of sufficient academic ability to cope with GCE 'O' and 'A' levels. The majority of these students showed no knowledge of mental handicap, had obviously never thought about it, and held views and expectations obviously based on the most extreme and bizarre degrees of subnormality. They expected that their parents would react adversely to the foundation of a hostel in their area, and justified this attitude by the supposed danger the mentally handicapped present to children and old people. Confusion between the mentally handicapped and the mentally ill was also very common.

Ignorance and prejudice are not confined to the populace at large but may readily penetrate the kin group. One of the South London mothers, for example, expressed a great deal of bitterness at the way the whole of her immediate family had suffered. They felt that they had been cut of from their wider family and from friends and the community:

> Let's put it this way, there were relations we have not seen since we found out about Trevor . . . [and] we have only been invited to tea with Trevor once to my brother-in-law. He thinks we should put Trevor away.

One justification for community care of mentally handicapped children, even if looking after them at home does lay a heavy burden on their mothers, is that they are thereby enabled to mix normally with other children and become assimilated into the normal life of the community. This was indeed a frequent outcome in our new city study, and where it occurs it forms an important and highly desirable part of the child's life. As with other children, not all make friends easily. In half of the families in our sample the children were described as 'not involved' with local children, or not interested in mixing with them, or in two cases as positively rejected by them, or else as having few opportunities to mix. (The 'mild' cases, surprisingly, seemed to be a trifle over-represented in this group.) In the other cases, however, neighbours and neighbouring children did play a very important part in the handicapped child's life. Involvement tends to be most intense, as one might expect, in small village communities:

> He chucks his wheelchair around the street and everyone knows him, he goes in next door and has an hour in there and a cup of tea and biscuits, and then he goes off down the road, the old people love him . . .
> . . .
> The wheel came off his wheelchair the other day, and a little tot . . . said 'Come quick, Edward's wheel has broken off his chair!' Well, I flew up . . . and there were these five little tots, none of them were more than six

(and he is a weight) and they had got it like this, and holding it so that he wouldn't go down. And their little faces! They really take care of him.

Urban life is also not incompatible with local involvement:

At the moment she's in love with the boy next door. He's sixteen and he's a nice lad, he takes an interest in her.

Even a blind and immobile child can benefit from local involvement:

[Her sisters'] friends come in and out. I think most of their friends are better with her than the grown-ups. Irene's . . . got a friend . . . orange hair one side and bright green the other . . . . If you saw her in the street you'd think, 'What a terrible child!' She'll come in here and she'll pick her up and she laughs and giggles and she's absolutely marvellous. But I find that all the teenagers and even younger . . . are very, very good. It's as they get to our age . . .

It is of course true, however, that the converse of assimilation will also occur, and the often adverse reactions which families experience from relatives and from the general public are one key definer of the world in which the mentally handicapped child lives. Reactions range from neutral or even highly support-ive (the latter particularly from the grandmothers of the children) to expres-sions of hostility, curiosity and distaste. One important point to note is that the parents of the mentally handicapped are of course themselves born mem-bers of the culture which despises their children, and they themselves carry these attitudes into their present situation. They may share them, or more likely fight them, or try to side-step them by aggressively declaring that their child is 'normal', but they cannot escape them; how they see their own situa-tion is shaped, positively or negatively, by cultural norms. Indeed, to bring the argument round full circle, the reactions which they perceive others as making may be supplied at least in part and on occasion by their own expectations. The point is well illustrated in an interview with one mother in the South London sample:

When I talk to people and I say, 'Mark is mentally handicapped', and as soon as they know he is coming up to sixteen, you see, you know what I mean? I don't want to put it into words, but you see it before they even say it. . . . It is an unspoken look. I suppose maybe I would be guilty in the same way, but there is that fear of danger to 'my daughter'.

However, even here the fact that the parents share, at some level, the same stigmatizing stereotype as they purport to recognize in others may be respon-sible at least in part for creating the problem – the parents may be over-sensitive, or may even project into the situation their own unacknowledged fears and feelings of distaste (see also Bayley, 1973, p. 240).

Thus having a mentally handicapped child and caring for him or her at home presents the child's parents with two major tasks which are not faced in the same way by parents of 'normal' children. They have to come to terms with the fact of the child's handicap and its implications for the way in which the family is able to conduct its normal life in interaction with others. At the same time they have to deal with the way our society labels and stigmatizes mental handicap – including the way that the historically determined stereotype of mental handicap spills over as a courtesy stigma for the whole family – and this means renegotiating the nature of the family's identity and building a style of life compatible with the renegotiated identity. This task is made none the easier by the fact that the parents are themselves members of the culture which stigmatizes them and their children, may project their own feelings of spoilt identity onto the world at large and share to some extent the very attitudes which they are forced to combat.

The mother's life

The work of community care, depite genuine assistance received in some cases from the family, the community and the state, tends to fall overwhelmingly on the mother. Similarly, despite the effects of handicap on the whole nuclear family which have been documented above, it is the mother's life and life opportunities which are most disrupted by having a mentally handicapped child. The extent of the burden will of course vary from family to family; very different lives and experiences are included under the one arbitrary label of mental handicap. When the children are very young they may not present a burden of care any greater than the norm, unless there are coexistent physical problems: 'children are wonderful anyway', and mongol babies and some of the mildly retarded are particularly quiet, sweet and undemanding as infants. The 'parenting style' adopted may not be very different from that considered appropriate for the other children in the family (which demonstrates how little the discoveries of educators and therapists percolate through to the family level – see Carr, 1975, p. 827). The degree of extra work may not be apparent to the mother herself because it has become 'just part of the routine'. In her survey of Scottish families, Hunter (1980) asked the question, 'How does having a handicapped child affect your family?' and received from one mother and answer, 'It's not until somebody asks you about it that you realise what you have to do.' We had a similar experience with our own research: an interim paper was discussed at a parents' meeting and the response to the section on the work of motherhood was that they had not realized until they saw it written out just how hard they did work. Nonetheless this labour and the need for it does exist, and the work falls predominantly on the child's mother.

Mothers of the mentally handicapped share with other mothers the substantial amount of work that bringing up any kind of child entails. The mentally handicapped child requires very much more labour over a lifetime, however. The work itself will generally be more intense. For example, all children are incontinent when they are young, but mentally handicapped children are incontinent for longer. Carr (1975) found that only 38 per cent of a sample of

Downs Syndrome children were 'clean and dry' by day by the age of four, and only 18 per cent by night, compared with 88 per cent and 71 per cent respectively of an age-matched control sample. In a survey of Family Fund applicants (Bradshaw, 1980) almost three quarters of the 242 children over the age of four were still incontinent. Even 'mild' cases may not be trained until they are four or five, and the most severely handicapped will be incontinent well into their teens, or for ever. This means not only more years of cleaning up and extra washing, but much more to clean up – as the child grows older – and a heavier child to manoeuvre on and off the pot. Disturbance at night may also be a normal feature of life for these families for many years beyond the normal, and there may be no ready escape from it.

Worries about supervision form a second major load on mothers. Bradshaw (1980) found that nearly half of the parents who applied to the Family Fund for assistance considered that their children were at risk of harming themselves or others if left alone for any period of time, and only 27 per cent felt the child could be left to play alone. We found the same kind of emphasis among the mothers to whom we spoke. The consequences are time diverted from housework and from the other children, and a consequent extension of the 'houseworking day', sometimes late into the evening. If the mother needs to go out, even just for shopping, the more intensive child care which mentally handicapped children often require may make it difficult to find baby-sitters or child-minders or to persuade relatives to share the care. (Even if it were not in fact more difficult, the parents may think that it would be, and that in itself is just as restricting.) Even when the children are at school the mother may need to remain 'on call', and timings have to be very precise, with very little leeway in the schedule – 'I mean, you can't really leave a handicapped child really on its own.' The child must be met from the school bus – in some cases the driver will not leave the child if there is no one there waiting. School times come to dominate the lives of such mothers even more tyranically than is normally the case:

> My life has been run by the school bus for fifteen years now. You can't go out; you must be here. From the day these children are born your life is planned; you've got to put it around that child.

In the holidays the child cannot be left even for half a day unsupervised, so school holidays are very likely to mean dropping all other activities to go back 'on guard'. Moreover, as the quotation above indicates, the process is protracted far beyond the norm. Many mothers would not leave their five-year-old child to come home from school to an empty house. Few, however, would still need to be there to receive a fifteen-year old, with the prospect of still needing to be there when the 'child' is twenty-five.

An important part of 'community care', as envisaged by its proponents, is the notion that 'the community' will support and sustain the family in its difficulties. Half of our new city sample did indeed receive considerable help from their neighbours, ranging from transport to hospital when needed or occasional baby-sitting to more crucial interventions. Two of the mothers were able to continue work when the children were still small because neighbours took care of them. Two more had neighbours on whom they could and did call in emergencies – for example, to meet the other children from school when the handicapped child had to be taken to hospital. One mother, indeed, was able to recruit a whole street of neighbours to apply an American training programme which calls for constant stimulation of the handicapped child. Eight families, however, did not know their neighbours or received little or no help from them. The kin-group, whether or not living in the immediate neighbourhood, was another important source of help or resources for some. Mothers, mothers-in-law, cousins and siblings provided money, transport for holidays, a warm place to take the baby from a cold flat, even the occasional 'weekend off'. Half of our sample, however, did not mention any degree of help from kin. In all, six of the sixteen received help from neither the people living round them nor from their wider family, and in another five cases the help they received was comparatively trivial.

Even the help which is received from the nuclear family is not enough to change mothers' burdens appreciably. Eight mothers in our study mentioned minor help delivered by the siblings of the handicapped child – domestic work, or minor help with child care, or in one case baby-sitting. One mother, a widow, received very substantial help from her eldest son. Among the fathers, five are described as helping with child-care – significant help in four cases. The contribution of six of them was not mentioned in either interview, which suggests they do as much or as little as most husbands. Five are described as doing little or nothing:

> Derek's not the sort of dad that does a lot, not knocking Derek, but I think he's an ideal man not to have kids . . .

> Harry has never been like a dad should be . . . He was very possessive, very possessive, but he never did anything to help me with him. I mean, he didn't walk till he was four. And never did he ever think of carrying him upstairs . . . well, he never done anything for him. That was a woman's job.

Thus some help is received from the surrounding community or from the kin group or indeed from within the nuclear family, but in general it is not enough to normalize the lives of the mothers who are caring for mentally handicapped children. Help from the family or from outside may carry one through an emergency or make mother's life easier or more pleasant. Nonetheless it is mother who bears the responsibility of care; others only 'help'. (Three of our mothers, indeed, mentioned no such help at all in either interview, and in two others the nuclear family was the only resource.)

Returning to a full-time job within a year or so of the birth is 'of course' out of the question for mothers of mentally handicapped children, as it appears to be for mothers of many 'normal' children (see next section). In our sample of sixteen mothers, for instance, none was currently in full-time paid employment, though all had worked before marriage. Seven had current employment of some sort – six in part-time or evening jobs, and one as a home-worker – and nine were not in employment at all. (Of this last group, however, two were already over sixty.) This kind of pattern of substantially less involvement with paid employment than is the norm even for other married women is borne out by a number of other studies (see, for example, Bayley, 1973; Glendinning, 1983). The inability to take full-time paid employment matters a great deal, because women work not only for the money (important though that may be) but also for the social contacts that 'going to work' brings and the increased social status which being engaged in paid employment brings in a society which devalues the domestic role.

Many of the reasons given for going down to part-time employment or giving up an outside job altogether in our study were such as might be given by any mother, whether or not her child was labelled as handicapped: the burden of child care, the need to be at home when the children come home from school, the difficulty of school holidays, the need to take leave when the children are ill. Some explicitly denied that the child's handicap was a factor. All but four had worked at some time since the birth of their children, in an occupation which fitted school hours: school canteen assistant was popular, as were part-time jobs in shops or offices (9 till 3.30), and some had worked evenings as a cleaner or on an assembly line. One or two had done child minding or short-term fostering, or run playgroups, and several had run 'Tupperware parties' and the like. One or two had managed a full-time job at some stage, but only because alternative child care was available. This kind of work pattern is fairly typical of any group of mothers. As we have seen, however, the mothers of the mentally handicapped have additional problems with which to contend.

People seem to be able to cope with almost anything, and most of our mothers coped with their load from day to day, trying to make a normal life for themselves and their families. One might want to distinguish, however, between families where 'normality' predominated and those where 'coping' is a more adequate descriptive term. In the latter class would fall those who would regard themselves as trying to treat the handicapped child as normal but who are resigned to the fact that they cannot entirely succeed in doing so and that the child makes a great deal of difference to their lives. They are 'resigned' to having a handicapped child rather than accepting of it, insofar as the two can be distinguished – they shade into each other. Often the problems lie with the nature of the handicap. Some children may be prone to violent outbursts, for example, out of frustration at their inability to communicate or, more worryingly, for no detectable reason. Sometimes the problem is to do with family lifestyle, as in the case of the busy mother who has three other children and manages to hold down an evening job as well when she is not child-minding or undertaking short-term foster care; the (mildly) handicapped child is just a cross which the family is resigned to bearing – loved and cared for, but a nuisance nonetheless. Sometimes a life which might have been comparatively easy is made difficult by the compounding pressure of other circumstances, as with Mrs Jones, a lady living on one of the rougher council estates, who appears from her own account and that of her husband to be suffering systematic persecution from a neighbouring family. In this 'coping' class we should also place 'Mrs Inglish', who is coping with life in general only with a great deal of social service support. Herself educated in a special school, and having spent a period in a psychiatric hospital, she has seldom held down a job for long; she is divorced, and the social services have assumed the parental responsibility for her children. Nonetheless, she is one who is managing to cope with the day-to-day care of the child.

One should remember that classifying a mentally handicapped child as 'the' problem of a family is a social construction which may not be shared by the family itself. For all the mothers we talked to the mentally handicapped child was indeed a problem, but for some there was another child about whom they worried more. Mrs Jones, for example, appeared more worried about her eldest child, who had a spell of truanting from school in response to the bullying from neighbouring children which followed on his evident grief at his grandmother's death. Another mother had a child suffering from cystic fibrosis who required daily medical or nursing attention. Another had a child who had been 'teacher's pet' at a small village school and was not reacting at all well to his transfer to a larger secondary school in the new city. Mrs Inglish was far more worried by her elder son Keith than by the mentally handicapped child; Keith is a boarder at a school for maladjusted children, and he tends to beat her up and smash the furniture when he comes home on holiday.

In four of our families 'adaptation' rather than just 'coping' might be said to have taken place: the child appears to play the same role in the family as a 'normal' child would do, and family life seems to proceed 'as normal'. (The distinction between this group and those who just cope is not a hard and fast one, however, and may be an artefact of what happened to 'come out' at particular interviews.) One middle-class lady who lived in one of the neighbouring villages, for example, used to work in an office until her child was born, went back to similar work when the child was three, and now (in her forties) does some work as a cook in the local school. She spends a great deal of time with her child and has to some extent 'built her life around her', but one has the impression that this would have been her pattern of life if the child had not been handicapped; she seems happy and settled. Another continued with part-time office work all the time she lived near relatives who could baby-sit, helped her husband for two years when he was running his own business, and is currently looking round for a part-time job which would involve her with children. She seems very close to and involved with both her children equally and to enjoy the life she has with them. Another lady with three children (one mildly retarded, and one with cystic fibrosis) presented herself in interview very much as a classic 'working-class mum'. She switched from full- to part-time factory work when she married, went over to working in the evenings when her first child was born, and switched again to cooking in a canteen when the others were born in order to be more available when they came out of school. The mentally handicapped child appears to have presented few problems once he was out of nappies and to be treated very much like her eldest, normal child. The fourth lady found she had to give up work to look after her children – apart from the odd cleaning job and running the occasional 'Tupperware party' – because her husband's long and irregular hours of work as a self-employed carpet fitter meant that he could not take regular responsibility for them. At the end of her interview, however, she surprised herself by saying:

> I think family life is important, and I mean, we are a normal family. My cousin said that once. I thought it was a queer thing to say. She said, 'I like it because you don't treat Edith anything but normal', and I said, 'Well, how the hell am I supposed to treat her?' But I thought about it afterwards and I suppose I could see what she meant, she wasn't being funny. We don't go out of our way because I've got a backward child, we don't not do anything, we do everything that, in fact, a normal family does.

These were all cases of a normal, unremarkable adaptation to family life. In six of our sixteen interviews, however, it is possible to detect a more exaggerated and systematic 'style' of adaptation. One mother, for instance, describes herself as very much enjoying married life and seeing children as an important and integral part of if. After school she worked in a shop, then took evening classes and became a clerk, but she gave up work when she 'fell for' her first child – a pre-marital but planned pregnancy. She has done odd jobs since – cleaning in the evenings, and lunch-time jobs – but she feels she could not take a settled job because of the handicapped child. However, she says she would not take a full-time job even if he were not there, because her other (older) child needs her at home. Another lady, Mrs Allinson, has not held a job since her handicapped daughter was born, and she very much enjoys not doing so; despite the amount of effort she puts into her life, she regards herself as something of a 'lady of leisure'. A third lady aspired to the same style. Talking of her early aspirations, she lists the chief one as 'just wanting to get married and have a family', and she says she looked forward to not working as a relief. However, she has found caring for her two chidren very hard work; only now that they both go out to school is she beginning to enjoy the leisure to which she had looked forward. The fourth started her working life in a factory, but she did not enjoy it and was glad to quit after she was married, when she 'fell for' her first child. She is beginning to think of taking some kind of part-time job, but that would be some considerable time in the future, as her oldest is only six.

These women might be seen, perhaps, as 'having marriage as a career' rather than just as being married. Another 'career' which one might detect in two of the interviews is that of child-minding. One lady, for example, had a family of five children spread over nine years and was then told she was very unlikely to be able to have any more. Eight years later, when she had supposed she was menopausal, she conceived 'by accident' and bore a severely brain damaged child. (She promptly had her seventh child, to provide him with company.) He is now sixteen, with an assessed mental age of about five but a 'social age' (we met him) which presents as very similar to his chronological age. She is now sixty, and he is very much the companion of her old age, while she is probably his closest friend and companion.

> He has been a marvellous child, he has given me lots and lots of plea-sure. . . . He'll stay. He won't be any different to what he is now. . . . By the time I do go . . . we're all long livers in my family . . . he'll have had a good life, as good as anyone could give him.

The second lady in this category says of herself that

> I've looked after young children all my life. I was always baby-minded, taking them out for walks. Very baby-minded person, when I was very young . . . that was my one aim in life, to have loads and loads of chil-dren. . . . I like children, you know, I like to be surrounded by children.

Of the 'respite' weekends that have been arranged for her, when Gerry goes into a hospital, she says

> It has taken me an awful long time to part with her even for odd weeks. . . . I didn't trust them, anyway, with her, to think that they could just automatically cope with her. So it's continuously on the 'phone every day, 'phoning up. It took me about – four she was the first time I let her go in – until eleven before I really knew who I was talking to.

That the reluctance to let her go was not just related to the quality of her care is emphasized later in the interview:

> Husband: You see, the first idea of relief care, whether it sounds harsh or not, was to get Lorna used to not having her around. . . . The idea in the beginning was to take her for longer and longer periods, so that she wouldn't be dependent on Gerry. You know, she wouldn't run her life.
> Wife: I think I should be lost without her: because my whole life does centre around her.

This case also provides a good illustration of how one's 'world picture' may change over time and how 'motivation' may sometimes be shaped teleo-logically to validate an outcome which is judged inevitable. At the time of our first interview she very definitely appeared to see herself as a child-centred person whose future employment would be in child care or in the care of the elderly – at least in part as a substitute for the daughter around whom her life had been centred until now. She confirmed in the second interview, a year later, that this had indeed been her picture of herself at the time and that she would indeed still feel lost and without purpose when Gerry has to go – that she might even break down at that point. However, since the first interview she had taken and passed a typing course and had every hope that she might obtain an office job at some time in the future if jobs of any kind were to be had. She now regards her earlier picture of her future as at least in part a rationalization of the inevitable.

In summary, the mother of the mentally handicapped child carries the same burden as any other mother – the burden of child care. This may be willingly accepted or even sought out and planned for, but it is nonetheless a life-consuming role which leaves little time or space for individuality. In that sense these mothers' lives are 'normal' for women, statistically and in terms of role-expectation, but as remote from the lives of men as are most married women's lives. Over and above the 'normal' constraints of other mothers, however, these women live a life more closely packed with problems, and the problems go on for a substantially longer period. This is the non-financial cost of community care.

Comparison with the 'normal'

Shortly after the second interviews with mothers of mentally handicapped children, one of us conducted a series of interviews with a 'sample' of mothers whose children had *not* been labelled as mentally handicapped, roughly matched for size of family and area of residence (which correlates well, in the new city, both with social class and with availability of 'social resources'). The sample is of course too small and haphazard to be representative of mothers in general – and a similar charge might be levelled at the sample of mothers of the mentally handicapped – but the two samples match closely enough for some tentative comparisons to be drawn. One can after all say little about what is distinctive in the experience of mothering mentally handicapped children except by comparison with the general experience of mothering.

Compared with our 'mental handicap' sample, very few of these mothers commented on the amount of work which having children around the house entails. Ten had no particular comment to make at all, except (in four cases) to say that they did not enjoy housework. Five, on the other hand, expressed positive pleasure in domestic work. For example:

> I'm just that kind of person, I like to be tidy. . . . I like to do everything . . . so that when I come home all I have to do really is tidy up in general down here, and give them a good cooked meal.
>
> (Mrs Blacker)

> People I know sit around and say 'I get bored', but I don't honestly get time. If I'm not gardening I'm decorating and if I'm not decorating I'm making – I do all my own dressmaking. If I'm not dressmaking I'm embroidering or knitting. Oh yes, I make the wine, I do the lot.
>
> (Mrs Greene)

> Washing their clothes, cooking for them, that's not hard work because it's a natural thing.
>
> (Mrs Royal)

Another lady described how she managed to render housework interesting by treating it as a nine-to-five job on the one hand and never letting it settle into an exact routine on the other. Only four people commented on the strains of the housewife's work, and their comments were to do mostly with how little sleep one seems to have during the first few years of a child's life.

One could well form the impression, in contradistinction to the mothers of mentally handicapped children, that these mothers did not regard the daily and yearly grind of motherhood as particularly hard work. This may to an extent be true: while mothering ordinary children is undoubtedly hard work, as anyone will testify who has children in the house, it is equally undoubtedly not as much work as mothering most mentally handicapped children. It differs in two other ways as well: (1) the children of these mothers were often of similar chronological ages to the children who appeared in the last section, but for this reason they were mostly more advanced in terms of development – the messier and heavier work lay in the past – and (2) the work entailed by a normal child has a forseeable termination, which often means that it seems less onerous. It may be also that mothers underrate the work of being a housewife precisely because it is 'normal', taken for granted by everybody concerned, while the mothering of a mentally handicapped child leads one to think about the work involved. Two other factors should also be considered, however. First, our sample underrepresents women in full-time paid employment, which could well make a difference – though the two women in our sample who were in full-time employment were not among the ones who commented on the pains of housework. The second factor is that the interviewer was male; it is possible that different things might have been said to a female interviewer.

As regards help with the work, we formed the impression from the interviews that the mothers of the unlabelled children received much the same help and support from kin, but more from neighbours, than did the mothers of the mentally handicapped children – that they were more closely integrated into the local community. Of the nineteen that we interviewed, twelve can be described as receiving (or having received in the past, when the children were younger) a fair amount of help from kin or neighours or both, and another two as having received occasional or emergency help. The parents and/or parents-in-law of six of the families lived in the neighbourhood, and four of them had received a good deal of help with child rearing or child care. One has a sister who takes the children overnight, and another a mother who advises and provides practical help (and nieces who baby-sit whenever required). Mrs Scarlett stayed with her mother for a few days after her second child was born, to give her time to recuperate while not interfering with her husband's ability to work. Another of these ladies would say that her family were not on the whole a great source of help, but her mother has been over once or twice a week during the current pregnancy, to do housework and ironing and anything else that she judged too much of a strain for a pregnant woman. Two others did not now see much of their parents, but they were a great source of help before they moved from London to the new city. For example, when Mrs Forrest's first child was a baby her husband's parents lived just round the corner, and her own were only seven miles away, so baby-sitting was never a problem and they were able to go out – in the evening or during the day – whenever they wanted to do so. (With her later children she has been more

restricted in that respect, but her parents come up for the weekend not infre-
quently, and Mrs Forrest and her husband generally take advantage of the
situation.) Six informants out of the nineteen rarely saw their parents or
received little help from them, and seven had little or nothing to say about kin,
but for six the 'extended family' was an important resource. This is much the
same picture as emerged from the analyses in the last section – round about a
third receiving significant help from the extended family.

A different picture emerges when we look at involvement with neighbours
and the local community. Eight of the mothers of mentally handicapped
children said they received little or no help from their neighbours, but only five
of the mothers of unlabelled children were in this position. Seven of the nineteen had a great deal of help from their neighbours – invaluable help in some
cases, making the desired lifestyle possible rather than impracticable.

> The neighbours are super.... I've always had a babysitter.... If I
> want to go to bed at ten in the morning and I've worked [on the night
> shift] the night before, my daughter gets her little shopping bag and goes
> off down [to a neighbour] . . . and goes with them to school. . . . You just
> couldn't do these things without neighbours.
>
> (Mrs Whiting)

Four others mentioned occasional help, and two help in emergencies. Overall
only five of the mothers of 'unlabelled' children had little or no help from either
kin or neighours, and twelve had a great deal of help from one or the other or
both. In comparison, eleven of the mothers of mentally handicapped children
received either no help at all or only trivial assistance.

As regards help from within the nuclear family, six of our informants'
husbands are described realistically (we checked by asking what they actually
did about the house) as taking a share or doing a great deal. For example:

> Whoever comes in first starts the dinner. You do the cooking [to her
> husband] and some of the cleaning. I think you have to, because we both
> go out now, doing different things.
>
> (Mrs Olivier)

> My husband does housework, he's tidier than I am, actually. The other
> night I was out. . . . I didn't get home till ten, and there he was ironing.
> He always bathes the kids. . . . He can cook dinner. I went to France on a
> day trip . . . and he had the children all day, and his Dad, he was out of
> hospital for the weekend . . . he cooked them a dinner and took them to
> the park.
>
> (Mrs Blacker)

> I suppose it's because I hate [housework] that they all do their bit, even
> the five year old does a bit around the house . . . The oldest boy cooks the
> dinner if ever we're not there. . . . [My husband] probably does more
> than I do, to be honest. I think he always has probably done more . . .
> because we've both always worked. . . . If it came to say who is really

> boss in the kitchen, he would be. . . . Two weeks out of three he does the shopping. . . . He probably taught me most of what I know about cooking anyway. . . . He'll do anything and everything around the house.
>
> (Mrs Whiting)

> I don't very often ask him to now, but when I had the children . . . he did ironing and different things. . . . If I'm not well . . . he'll just come in and take over. When we were first married and both working, he'd come in and maybe wash up while I hoovered and things like that.
>
> (Mrs Forrest)

Another lady described how her husband will take over getting the supper and send her up to have a bath, when he gets in from work, if he thinks she looks under the weather, and how he has done her evening cleaning job once or twice when she has been ill. Seven others describe their husbands as doing a bit about the house – child care (3) or housework (1) or both (3) – but only in the sense of 'helping'. Six others described their husbands as offering little or no daily help. Adding these in, this still leaves three families where the wife receives virtually no help in keeping up the house and looking after the children, from nuclear family or kin or neighbours. The same number were without help in the families with mentally handicapped children.

Overall, then, the mothers of the unlabelled children and the mothers of the mentally handicapped children had much the same resources to draw on in their 'home work', with the exception that the mothers of unlabelled children seemed to receive more help from the surrounding community. One should not overrate the amount or quality of the help, however, in the majority of cases. While a few of our informants praised their husbands for the amount of work they did around the house and/or with the children, in only two cases were they prepared to say that the husband did as much (or more) as they did themselves, or that they could relinquish responsibility for the work. This is the general finding of research into husbands' involvement in the work of the home. Men may on occasion be substantially involved in child care – and perhaps increasingly so – but seldom in the remaining work of the house (though if mothers are asked not which tasks the husband undertakes but how often he undertakes them or how many hours he spends on them, it turns out that nearly fifty per cent of married men with children can best be described as only minimally involved in child care – see Boulton, 1983). As regards housework, Edgell's 1980 study suggests that virtually no husbands take an equal share, and nearly half do virtually none. The families whom we have interviewed do not seem to be as extreme – there were a few cases of genuine help, within the limitation of work constraints – but we also formed the impression that most women nonetheless receive precious little help in the day-to-day running of the house, and certainly that the running of the house remains the woman's responsibility in the vast majority of cases.

In this context, Backett (1982) has pointed out in relation to her study of couples in an Edinburgh suburb that:

> In order for couples to sustain belief in [high] levels of father involvement
> they did not see it as necessary for him to participate fully or constantly.
> Rather it is a matter of each couple negotiating the kind of practical
> proof which they found to be subjectively satisfactory. This was done by
> the father's participating sufficiently regularly in those particular spheres
> which spouses had identified as being relevant to their own family
> situation.

(p. 221)

She also points out that the situation for men is fundamentally different from
the situation for women, where the man goes out to work and the wife stays at
home. When the husband is at home, even if he were literally to take an equal
share of available 'home work', it is a share; his wife is there to carry the other
half. Thus a man may 'do' child care, or housework, and be fully committed to
it. Never or seldom, however, is he faced with the daily problem that his wife
faces when he is not at home – that both housework and child care have to be
coped with at one and the same time.

In the sample of sixteen mothers of mentally handicapped children,
described in the last section, none was in full-time paid employment at the time
of the interview. Six were in part-time or evening jobs, one was a home
worker, and nine were not working at all. Of our sample of nineteen mothers
whose children were not labelled as mentally handicapped, two were in full-
time employment (a proportion which undoubtedly underrates the proportion
in the population – those we approached who were in full-time employment
tended to decline the interview), six were in a substantial part-time job, two
did some part-time paid work and some voluntary work, one was substantially involved in voluntary work (as a WI county organizer), and three others
did a small amount of part-time work or home work and helped out at their
children's schools. Only five were in no form of employment, and one of those
was in a late stage of pregnancy. The two groups differ substantially on this
variable, therefore: the mothers of mentally handicapped children were
markedly less able to take outside employment.

However, we should note that the presence of children in the home still
made a substantial difference to the pattern of employment. Of those who
worked full-time, one was on the night shift (as a nurse) so that there was
always someone in the house to look after the children. Of the eight who were
in part-time employment, six had jobs deliberately chosen to leave them free to
be home when the children came home from school (morning work in a garage
office, day-time shifts as a nurse, or the jobs in canteens or as school welfare
officers which are so popular with mothers). There were no cases of men
similarly curtailing their work patterns in the interests of the children. The
responsibility for the children's welfare still falls disproportionately on the
mothers.

Other factors which were evident in the 'mental handicap' interviews were
far less salient in the other ones. Mothers of mentally handicapped children
talked a great deal about the difficulties of being tied to the timetable of the

child, which was a minority response among the other mothers interviewed; the unlabelled children remained children in that sense for a much shorter period before they could be trusted to look after themselves to some limited extent. The initial adaptation to the child was of course a major theme in the interviews with mothers of mentally handicapped children and not in the others, though there were a few comments about the difficulty of adapting to the lack of freedom (and of sleep!) which young children entail. Most noticeable was the relative absence in the interviews with mothers of unlabelled children of comments about the longer-term adaptations which the family had undergone and of the family's plans for the future. It seemed taken for granted in the majority of cases that having children was a temporary phase, though of long duration, yet on the other hand there was relatively little conscious planning for the future. One had the impression more of a state of faith that the future would take care of itself in a relatively unproblematic way, 'as it does for everybody else'.

The family's future

'In the normal course of things' children grow from babies to toddlers, go to school and become increasingly independent in their lives, they leave school, find a job (or, increasingly, fail to do so) and eventually cease to be the responsibility of their parents. As we have seen, mentally handicapped children generally go through the early stages of this life-course more slowly than others and thereby create substantial burdens which generally fall on their mothers. In their adolescence, however, they may constitute a substantial problem for both parents, because for some of them there is every likelihood that they will never leave home at all unless their parents make specific arrangements to send them away. As Dickerson and Brown (1978) have pointed out, the parents.

> . . . have one child who is not going to release them from responsibility. It gets to be a very big worry. Who is going to support this child? Who will pay the bills? Provide him a good home? Supervise his leisure time . . .? Keep him out of trouble . . .? The parents find that they need to make long-term arrangements for the disabled child in the event of their deaths.

In the shorter term, the children leave school at some time in their teens and may therefore no longer be 'off their parents' hands' during the day.

One of the problems is that handicapped children grow less wonderful as they grow older. What was acceptable appearance and behaviour in someone who looks five or ten years old may no longer be acceptable in someone who looks twenty or thirty. Several of the mothers in the South London sample commented on this problem, and one had even had her daughter institutionalized to avoid the expected problems:

This is one reason why something would have to be done. She went into the hospital . . . when she was 21. Caroline was 3 and Michael was 19, coming up to 20. I have seen so many families where the brothers have girlfriends and this causes unpleasantness, and . . . I said we have got to do something before Michael starts going serious with girlfriends, before Caroline goes to school and brings friends home. We don't want to make any unpleasantness.

At the same time, the mentally handicapped child may paradoxically become relatively younger – more of a burden to the family – in proportion as he or she becomes older physically. Even if no more of a burden, the 'child' remains the same burden for year after year in a 'frozen' family which has lost the space to change and in which the parents themselves are becoming older and less able to cope.

While the family's development is frozen, however, social provision is not: the provision for a family with a handicapped child tends if anything to decline as the 'child' grows past school age. The real 'community care' for mentally handicapped children who grow into mentally handicapped adults is that they follow the 'normal' pattern and leave home – for a hostel and sheltered work, for a farm community or a group home, or for a hospital. For most families the time when children leave home is in any case a 'crisis point', but for the families of the mentally handicapped it is likely in addition to involve great feelings of guilt, because the child is generally not leaving home 'naturally' but being 'pushed out'. In the sixteen families we interviewed in the new city, only one mother saw her retarded child as likely to leave home and live a normal life; this was a mildly handicapped child of fourteen who was already showing every sign of being able to cope adequately and whose retarded uncles were coping in the outside world. Six others thought their child would always stay at home with them, but half of these were also considering the possibility of placement in a hostel or a sheltered community when they became unable to cope. Two (whose children were aged respectively eight and five) had not considered the topic. The other seven were already beginning negotiations for a hostel place or a place in a resdential school or community. Thus well over half of our sample had to deal in their minds with the possibility or the likelihood of handing care over to others, and of these seven were expecting or fearing that the care would have to be in some sort of institution. The very childishness which makes the child a burden at home and necessitates the arrangements for continuity of care, paradoxically, increases the stress and the guilt of relocation:

When you think what her mental age is, say four or five, by the time she's nineteen it won't be much more than that. You wouldn't stick a five-year old in a hostel, would you?

The choice of a proper institution or facility and the battle to be accepted there – as funds, and therefore places, are limited – can be a problem before which all earlier problems seem trivial and manageable.

Conclusions

To recapitulate, then, we have looked in this paper at the real costs of bearing and bringing up a mentally handicapped child in the community. Some of it – the day-to-day grind of 'child work' – falls largely on the child's mother, though her involvement in it has consequences for the rest of the family. The rearing of a mentally handicapped baby does not differ in kind from the rearing of any other baby – itself a substantial social burden – but it differs in its density and its duration. The care of a retarded child may require constant vigilance, and the lateness of normal 'stages of development' doubles or trebles the burden of an 'ordinary' problem such as incontinence. The burden goes on, moreover, potentially for ever, unless the decision is made to send the child away – to the point where aging parents can no longer cope or provision must be made for what happens after their death or in the case of their eventual incapacity. (The potential exceptions – at least three out of our sample of sixteen – are those whose children are not expected to live beyond their twenties; some of the mental handicaps have coexistent physical problems of great severity.) Specific to mental handicap, however, are the other major range of problems which families encounter: the reactions which the notion of mental handicap engenders in our culture, among strangers and also within the family and kin group. Not least of this range of problems is that the parents of the retarded are themselves a part of the culture which stereotypes retardation and have to cope with their own reactions and their expectations of how others will react as well as with the real situation.

References

Abbott, P. A. (1982). *Towards a Social Theory of Mental Handicap*. PhD thesis, Thames Polytechnic.

Backett, K. C. (1982). *Mothers and Fathers: A Study of the Development and Negotiation of Parental Behaviour*. Macmillan, London.

Bayley, M. (1973). *Mental Handicap and Community Care*. Routledge & Kegan Paul, London.

Birenbaum A. (1970). On managing a courtesy stigma. *Journal of Health*, 196–206.

Boulton, M. G. (1983). *On Being a Mother: A Study of Women with Pre-School Children*, Tavistock, London.

Bradshaw, J. (1980). *The Family Fund: An Initiative in Social Policy*. Routledge & Kegan Paul, London.

Carr, J. (1975). *Young Children with Down's Syndrome: Their Development, Upbringing and Effects on their Families*. Butterworth, London.

Cummings, S. T. (1976). The impact of the child's deficiency on the father: a study of fathers of mentally retarded and chronically ill children. *American Journal of Orthopsychiatry*, 46, 246–255.

Dickerson, M. and Brown, S. (1978). A search for a family. In S. Brown and M. Moersch (eds), *Parents on the Team*. University of Michigan Press, Michigan.

Edgell, S. (1980). *Middle-Class Couples: A Study of Segregation, Domination and Inequality in Marriage*. Allen & Unwin, London.

Gallagher, J. J, Beckman, P. and Cross, A. H. (1983) Families of handicapped children: sources of stress and its amelioration. *Exceptional Children*, 50, 10–19.

Glendinning, C. (1983). *Unshared Care: Parents and their Disabled Children*. Routledge & Kegan Paul, London.

Goffman E. (1963). *Stigma: the Management of Spoilt Identities*. Penguin, Harmondworth.

Greengross, W. (1976). *Entitled to Love?* Marriage Guidance Council, London.

Hunter, A. B. J. (1980). *The Family and their Mentally Handicapped Child*. Barnardo Social Work papers no. 12.

Shearer, A. (1972). *A Report on Public and Professional Attitudes Towards the Sexual and Emotional Attitudes of Handicapped People*. Spastics Society/National Association for Mental Handicap, London.

Tredgold, A. F. and Soddy, K. (eds) (1970). *Tredgold's Mental Retardation*, 11th ed. Baillière, Tindall & Cox, Eastbourne.

Walker, N. and McCabe, S. (1973). *Crime and Insanity in England*, vol. II. University of Edinburgh Press, Edinburgh.

## 5

Planning research: A case of heart disease

Pamela Abbott

This chapter is concerned to explain how I and a colleague (Geoff Payne) made the decisions which we did make about the design and sample size for a survey that we are carrying out in collaboration with a District General Hospital in the South-West of England. Issues of research design and sampling are crucial to the credibility of the research findings. Mistakes and misjudgements made at this stage of the research programme are difficult if not impossible to rectify at a later stage. Textbooks on research methods tend to lay down definitive statements about research designs and sample sizes, while our own theoretical perspectives may lead us to prefer one style of research to another. However, as I shall show here, both theoretical preferences and textbook ideals have to be compromised when we are confronted with the 'real world' and are actually carrying out research in it. It is also essential to recognize that when research is commissioned the researcher is being employed as an expert in research. Those commissioning the research may have a political agenda, which may or may not be shared by the researcher. Provided the researcher does not have ethical objections to the purpose of the research, however, politics have to be kept outside the planning and conduct of the research. Just as we may believe such and such a hypothesis to be true but be required as researchers to design a study which allows the possibility that the hypothesis can be disproved, so we may hold a political position and have hopes for the outcome of a piece of research but are required to design it to allow the possibility that the opposite position could be upheld by it.

The request for us to undertake research was made by the consultant cardiac surgeon at a District General Hospital. He approached the Faculty of Human Sciences at Polytechnic South West, to explore the possibility of collaborative research. The design of the research, sampling and sample size were discussed fully with him at all stages of the planning process.

The specific problem which he wanted researched was the experiences of patients who had to travel to East London for open-heart surgery. The District General Hospital has no facilities for such surgery, and all patients, private and national health, have to travel to London. The journey time by public transport to the hospital in London is at least five hours for these patients, and considerably longer for those who live in the rural areas surrounding the urban area where the District General Hospital is located. The initial problem with which we were asked to assist was the investigation of how patients and their partners actually experienced the travel to and the stay in London. It was hoped that this would provide a basis for developing better ways of preparing patients and partners, and specifically that it would enable a booklet to be written that could be given to all patients referred to London. However, it quickly became evident that the consultant had a 'hidden agenda': he was obviously interested in obtaining evidence to use in a campaign to procure open-heart surgery provision at the District General Hospital, and he hoped the research would begin to provide a basis for evaluating patients' experiences of 'internal markets' within the NHS. For this reason we tried to design the research so that our politics did not influence the research process or dictate the outcomes.

The design of the research and the decisions on sampling size emerged over a period of time, as we became aware of the complex nature of the issues with which we were dealing. Initially I felt that this was a research area that necessitated a qualitative approach. My preference at this stage was for in-depth interviews with patients and their partners to explore in detail their experiences and to find out what additional help they would find beneficial. This would have enabled us to explore in depth how people actually experienced travelling to London. It would have given us a vivid picture of what happened, what they experienced and how they felt about it. An informal, naturalistic interview procedure would have encouraged them to provide frank and detailed information. However, the costs of such methods, in time and the small number of people that could be interviewed, made them impractical. We could have handled only a small sample of couples, and this may well have provided atypical accounts; we needed 'across-the-board' information to provide a basis for helping future patients and their partners. We therefore decided that we would design a questionnaire, with analysis being undertaken using SPSSx on computer. We tried to keep the questions as naturalistic as possible, however; that is, the questions dictate the subject matter of the response but do not delimit the range of responses. Given the wide geographical area from which patients travel to the District General Hospital, we thought at this time that we would use a postal questionnaire.

In order to design the questionnaire we decided that we needed to know more about the actual experience of patients and their partners. The consultant cardiac surgeon arranged for four former patients (two male and two female) who had travelled to London for surgery, and their partners, to come to the District General Hospital. Geoff Payne and I carried out an open-ended group interview, which was taped and transcribed. This was used to provide basic information for the design of the questionnaire. Drafts of the two questionnaires, one for patients and one for their partners, were sent out to these six people, and they were asked to complete them, to suggest any questions that they thought we should have asked and to give their comments. Copies of the questions we asked were also sent to the consultant and the ward sister on the cardiac unit for their comments. On the basis of their comments the questionnaires were amended. It also became evident that it would not be possible to use them as postal questionnaires, given the difficulties these patients reported in completing the questionnaires at home themselves, but that an interviewer would be needed. It was agreed that interviews could take place at the hospital when the patients were asked to come in for a routine examination.

The analysis of the transcribed material and consideration of what we wanted to find out – which was now a broader range of questions than just what was needed to compile an information booklet – also led us to realize that it was not sufficient to interview patients and their partners who had already been to the London hospital. First, it became evident that we needed to follow a sample of patients and their partners through the process – that is, to interview them before they went to London and after they or their partner had undergone surgery in London. This would enable us to gain a much better understanding not only of how people felt about the process and their actual experiences but also of the types of information and support that could be given. It was also evident from the transcribed group interview that we needed to separate out the specific problems and difficulties associated with travelling to London from their experience of undergoing a major operation which was perceived to be life-threatening, or of being the partner of such a person. We realized that we needed a comparison or control group. Ideally this group should be identical to our sample except that they or their partners did not have to travel a long distance to have surgery. The obvious choice initially would seem to be the local patients at the London hospital. However, on reflection we realized that not only would it be practically difficult for us in terms of carrying out the interviews, but the characteristics of the London population were very different from those of our South-West sample of England. This precluded that possibility of a time-constrained sample of all patients (which is what we were using as the South-West sample). It might have been possible to use a matched-pair design – selecting a patient in London who had the same characteristics as each patient from the South-West. However, this would have extended the length of the study by an unknown amount, and the London sample would of course have been untypical of London patients. A further complication was that we did not have the same facilities in London as we had negotiated in the District General Hospital to interview patients. We decided that we would have to use, as a comparison, patients who were treated at the local hospital who were undergoing a procedure of a similar nature and were likely to have comparable characteristics. The consultant cardiologist suggested that patients undergoing major aortic repair would be suitable in terms of the cirteria we specified.

This meant we now had a research design that involved us in interviewing six groups of people:

1. Patients who had undergone heart surgery in London.
2. The partners of these patients.
   These were retained in the design, although formally redundant because the information is duplicated by Groups 3 and 4, because we needed data to get the information booklet out as quickly as possible, given that a before-and-after design takes considerably longer than retrospective research. In this case patients may have to wait some time between referral to the hospital in London and the actual date of the operation. We would then have to allow them to return from London and recover (at least six weeks) before they were interviewed.
3. Patients who were referred for heart surgery to London (to be interviewed when first told of the referral, and after the operation).
4. The partners of such patients (also to be interviewed twice, at the same points).
5. Patients undergoing aortic repair at the District General Hospital (again interviewed before and after).
6. The partners of such patients.

The questionnaires for the six groups were designed on the basis of responses to the first two that had been developed and piloted. The coding frame for the analysis of the data when the interviewing was completed was developed at this stage as well. When the questionnaires for Groups 1–4 were prepared, we trained the interviewer. She then carried out a small number of interviews at the hospital, and on the basis of feedback from her, some minor modifications were made to the questionnaires. The six final versions were prepared and printed, using a different colour of paper for each questionnaire.

The other key issue was sample size. We wanted a large enough sample to be able to analyse the data using two- and three-way tables – to be able to display the interaction of one variable with another taking account of a third (i.e. differences between partners and patients in terms of worries about the operation, controlling for social class or for age of patient), and to use a test of significance such as Chi-squared to check that the results were not likely to be random sampling variations. We also wanted, for the retrospective groups (Groups 1 and 2), to collect the information reasonably soon after the operation, because of the risk of memory loss or distortion. Given the reasons for the research we did not want it to extend over more than two years, including data collection, analysis and report writing. We also wanted the sample to be representative of people undergoing open-heart surgery in the area (a quite diverse group, as it turned out). About 200 NHS patients are referred from the area each year to the hospital in East London for open-heart surgery. (We excluded private patients because of the small numbers and because they are referred to a different London hospital.) We decided that this gave us an adequate sample size and fitted in with our timing. We would interview all patients who had undergone open-heart surgery in the previous twelve months and all those referred to London in the coming twelve months. A similar-sized sample of aortic repair patients would be interviewed at the same time.

So we had designed our research and decided on our sample size. Two additional elements were added at this stage. We decided that a simple stress questionnaire would be administered by a nurse as part of the routine procedures on admission to hospital for surgery – both for those in London who were going to have open-heart surgery and those in the District General Hospital who were having surgery to repair the aortic artery. This would enable us to determine if those patients travelling to London for major surgery showed more evidence of stress than those having surgery at the local hospital. We also decided that a researcher would travel to London on public transport with a small subset of the open-heart patients, to observe and to talk to them and the people travelling with them. This would give some qualitative data on how patients and their partners actually experienced the journey and being admitted to the hospital or finding accommodation convenient to it.

The research was designed so that we could provide information, when the data were collected, on the experience of travelling to London for surgery, the problems that people experienced and how they felt about it all. It was also designed so that we could determine what factors were attributable to travelling and what to the fact that the patient was about to have major surgery. It was aimed both at providing this information and to act as a basis for helping patients and partners to be better prepared and supported by the hospital staff in the South when they had to travel to London for surgery. At the point at which this chapter was written, field work had only just begun. However, the specific outcomes we expect are:

1. A practical booklet for patients and their partners, explaining to them what will happen and giving useful information.
2. Providing advice to nurses and doctors on how they can better prepare patients travelling to London for heart surgery (and possibly more generally to nurses and doctors caring for any patients who have to travel some distance for treatment).
3. Contributing to the debate on internal markets in the NHS.

## 6

Hospital visiting on two wards

Pamela Abbott and Geoff Payne

Introduction and background to the research

This report summarizes the results of research commissioned by the Plymouth Community Health Council (PCHC) from the Department of Applied Social Science, Polytechnic South West, into visiting on the gynaecological and maternity wards of Freedom Fields/Greenbank Hospital, Plymouth. At the request of the PCHC, the Plymouth Health Authority introduced open visiting at the Authority's hospitals in 1986. In practice this means that on a majority of the wards visitors are permitted between 2.00 p.m. and 8.00 p.m. The intention was that visitors would be able to come at any time between these hours, giving greater flexibility in choice of times at which to visit. The nurses on the maternity unit at Freedom Fields/Greenbank Hospital approached the PCHC, suggesting that the new visiting arrangements were unsatisfactory. They argued that insufficient time was left for carrying out necessary nursing duties and for mothers to learn how to handle their new babies. It was also said that the mothers found the new arrangements tiring.

When we made preliminary visits to the nursing officer in charge of the hospital's maternity unit, and to the wards, we found a somewhat different set of conditions. On the one hand, the nurses had developed several unofficial (or 'informal') rules that modified the basic official (or 'formal') visiting regulations, and made them easier to work. For example, there was in practice considerable flexibility in the times at which visitors were allowed. Partners and mothers, in particular, were allowed to visit outside the official hours. Requests for others to visit outside the official hours were also frequently sympathetically received.

The formal rules on numbers were also not rigidly enforced, despite expressed concern that more than two people were visiting some patients at the same time. The nurses' concerns could be more narrowly focussed on to three specific problems. These were:

(a) the length of time that visitors stayed – that is, some visitors felt that they had to stay for the whole of the visiting period;

(b) the numbers of visitors who were neither close relations nor friends coming to see the new baby (with the suggestion that some of these people would not have been welcomed in the mother's own home);

(c) disruption caused by visiting by young children.

While it was recognized that a mother's own children should be free to visit her, it was felt that other young chilren should not be allowed. Although some effort had been made to enforce the rules on children other than the patients' *not* being allowed to visit, it was felt to be difficult to do so once visitors had arrived accompanied by the children.

The gynaecological wards were selected as a 'control group'. The nurses on these wards had not contacted the PCHC. However, it was felt that these wards were likely to have some of the same problems (especially children visiting and excessive lengths of stay) but not others (such as excessive numbers of non-close visitors). Also, these wards were likely to have patients who were very unwell alongside those who had undergone only minor operations. The majority of new mothers are not seriously ill, although they may be tired immediately after the birth.

We did not speak to the gynaecological staff prior to carrying out the research. However, after the patient and visitor interviewing had been carried out, one of us (P.A.) spent a couple of days in one of the gynaecological wards. This enabled her to carry out informal interviewing of staff and some participant observation, which revealed that as on the maternity wards there were informal rules and a degree of flexibility in the enforcement of rules. On admission, patients were told that visiting was from 2.00 p.m. to 5.00 p.m. and from 6.00 p.m. to 8.00 p.m. – the period from 5.00 p.m. to 6.00 p.m. being when patients had their evening meal. (P.A. was told by the nursing staff, however, that if visitors who turned up during this period had travelled some distance or could not wait until later, they would be admitted.) The patients certainly preferred not having visitors watch them eating their evening meal. The staff also felt that there was a problem with visitors staying an excessive time, with the numbers visiting, and with visiting by young children. However, they said that the problem of numbers was relatively minor.

The study

Methods

Three separate questionnaires were developed for visitors, patients, and nurses. The first two of these were prepared by a group of second year BA(Hons) Social Policy and Administration students under the direction of the authors. These questionnaires were piloted in December 1986, and the interviews on which this report is based were carried out by students in January–March of 1987. The nurses' questionnaire was drawn up later and sent to the maternity nurses in May 1987 and to the gynaecological nurses in July. It was designed for self-completion. Anonymity was guaranteed to all who participated in the research.

The sample

The samples of visitors and patients were originally intended to be time-limited but exhaustive – that is, interviewing was to be carried out over a two-week period at whatever time of day the students could manage and every visitor or patient was to be approached until each student had obtained a predetermined number of interviews. However, two weeks proved to be too short a time for the collection of a large enough sample, and interviewing was continued over a longer period. Each student was asked to interview eight patients and eight visitors, but this proved impossible for some students, given the 'turn-round' on pre-natal and gynaecological wards. Students carried out interviews during normal visiting hours, each ward being allocated to two or three students. Visitors were approached as they arrived and asked if they would be prepared to answer a few questions, then or later. The large majority of those approached agreed. Patients were selected in advance by nursing staff so that students did not approach those felt to be too ill to participate, or cause embarrassment to those who would prefer not to do so. Visitors and patients had to be interviewed on the wards. In all, 88 visitors and 90 patients were interviewed.

All the nurses on both Units were sent a self-completion questionnaire and asked to return it in an envelope provided. The response was disappointingly low, five completed questionnaires being received from nurses working on the gynaecological wards and seventeen from the maternity unit.

Results

The visitors

General characteristics A total of 88 visitors to the hospital were interviewed; of these, one was visiting a ward not included in the survey. Sixteen of those interviewed were visiting gynaecological wards, and sixty maternity wards. Forty-one (47%) of the visitors interviewed were male. Ages varied from 15 years to over 65 years, with a high concentration in the 25–34 age-band as would be expected from the age of the patients on maternity wards. Of the visitors interviewed, the majority were coming to see a relative (87.5%). The remainder were, with one exception, visiting a 'close friend', so that even where the person being visited was a neighbour the relationship was seen as close.

Just under half of the visitors came alone. The majority of those who were accompanied came with either one or two other people. The overwhelming majority (87%) of these other visitors were family. Visitors were accompanied by a relatively small number of children, eight boys and thirteen girls in all, and no group of visitors included more than two children. Seventeen of the visitors were accompanied onto the ward by the children, one child stayed for only part of the visit, and one child did not go onto the ward.

Visiting problems and numbers of visitors   Visitors seem to have experienced few problems in their visiting. Only seven said they had been asked to leave the ward on that day or on a previous occasion. Most of these had been asked to leave by a nurse 'for medical reasons', or because the patient was to be examined, or in one case for unspecified reasons.

The number of visitors which any patient received seemed to exceed the number allowed. On the day the interview took place, 35 (49%) of the patients being visited had two visitors or fewer, according to the visitors, while 37 (51%) had more than the permitted number. However, only six (7%) of the visitors thought that there had been too many visitors. No-one thought that three visitors were too many, and two of the three people visiting patients with eight or more visitors did *not* think that this was too many. It was argued that in general patients liked visits. However, those that felt there were too many visitors on this occasion gave as their reason that it was too much of a strain for the patient or that the patient was tired.

Again, when visitors were asked about the number of visitors on other occasions the number per patient was not found to be too large; indeed, there had only been one visitor on previous occasions in 87 per cent of cases, and only in ten per cent of cases had the official numbers been exceeded even once. There is also no evidence from these answers of large numbers of visitors to *other* patients on previous occasions.

In conclusion, visitors are happy in general with the arrangements for visiting and the provisions made for it on the gynaecological and maternity wards at Freedom Fields/Greenbank Hospital. There is little evidence that children or excessive numbers of visitors are perceived by other visitors as causing a nuisance, nor is there general dissatisfaction with visiting hours. However, visitors certainly want more than two visitors per patient to be permitted and do not think that the rules should be strictly enforced.

The patients

General characteristics   Ninety female patients were interviewed; 63 (70%) were on maternity wards, and 27 (30%) on gynaecological wards. The length of time that they had been in hospital ranged from less than three days (37%) to more than one month (1%). The largest number had been in for between three and seven days (see Table 6.1). The majority of the patients admitted had come in for childbirth (43%); 12 (13%) had come in for bed-rest during pregnancy, nine (10%) for a hysterectomy/Manchester repair, and five (6%) for a 'D and C'.

Most of the patients interviewed were visited regularly. However, fewer patients on the gynaecological wards were visited at least once a day than on the maternity wards. Seven (25%) of the patients on the gynaecological wards were visited less than once a day, compared with only one woman on the maternity wards (see Table 6.2). Seventy-nine (88%) were visited by their husbands, and 87 per cent of these husbands visited regularly. Just over half (59%) of the patients were visited by their mothers, but only about half of these mothers were regular visitors. Thirty-seven (41%) were visited by their own children, of whom about 60 per cent were regular visitors. Only a small number were visited by neighbours (7%) and children other than their own (10%). Full details are given in Table 6.3.

Visiting problems and numbers of visitors The patients were asked the greatest number of visitors they had received and the largest number of children visiting at one time for each day out of the previous seven. (Obviously some of them had not been in hospital for the whole of this period.) This produced no evidence of excessively large numbers of visitors or of large numbers of children visiting, although a very small group of patients did have large groups of visitors (see Tables 6.4 and 6.5).

Table 6.1 Type of ward and length of stay of patients

Type of ward	Length of stay			
	< 3 days	3 to < 7 days	≤ 1 month	> 1 month
Maternity	29 (46%)	25 (40%)	8 (13%)	1 (1%)
Gynaecology	4 (15%)	16 (59%)	7 (26%)	–
Total	33 (37%)	41 (46%)	15 (17%)	1 (1%)

Table 6.2 Type of ward and frequency of visits

Type of ward	Frequency of visits	
	Once or more per day	Less than once per day
Maternity	62	1
Gynaecology	20	7
Total	82 (91%)	8 (9%)

Table 6.3 Relationship and regularity of visitors

Relationship to patient	n	Percentage	Percentage of these who were regular visitors
Husband	79	87.8	87.3
Mother/Mother in Law	53	58.9	52.8
Own children	37	41.1	59.5
Father/Father in Law	27	30.0	48.1
Other relatives	33	36.7	24.2
People from work	10	11.1	30.0
Other children	9	10.0	22.2
Neighbours	6	6.7	50.0

Table 6.4 Greatest number of visitors (in percentages)

Number	Yesterday (Day 1)	Day before (Day 2)	Day 3	Day 4	Day 5	Day 6	Day 7
0	13.3	44.4	57.8	65.6	77.8	82.2	86.7
1	18.9	24.4	14.4	12.2	11.1	4.4	4.4
2	31.3	13.3	12.2	15.6	5.6	10.0	6.7
3	18.9	11.1	8.9	4.4	5.6	2.2	1.1
4	8.9	4.4	4.4	2.2	–	1.1	1.1
5	5.6	2.2	–	–	–	–	–
6–9	3.3	–	2.2	–	–	–	–

Table 6.5 Greatest number of children visiting (in percentages)

Number	Yesterday (Day 1)	Day before (Day 2)	Day 3	Day 4	Day 5	Day 6	Day 7
0	67.8	83.3	83.3	88.9	90.0	91.1	93.3
1	20.0	11.1	7.8	6.7	6.7	5.6	3.3
2	7.8	4.4	5.6	4.4	1.1	3.3	1.1
3	–	1.1	1.1	–	–	–	–

A large majority of the patients (71–79%) liked the present arrangements; although the percentage liking them was higher on the gynaecological wards than on maternity wards (89% as compared with 76%), the difference is not statistically significant.

The patients also felt they had about the right number of visitors. Seventy-eight (87%) said the number they had was about right, four (4%) thought they had too many, and seven (8%) would have liked more. (No differences between types of ward or between those who liked or disliked the present arrangements were detected.) The main reason given by those who felt they had too many visits was that they found them tiring, while those who had too few said they found the long day boring. A small number named people who they would prefer *not* to visit them. Two of these mentioned children, one because the child got restless and the other because the child was noisy. Four mentioned relatives who they did not want to visit, and a further nine mentioned another unspecified person, the reason given being that they 'did not get on'.

Again, most of the patients (83%) felt that their visitors stayed for about the right length of time. However, seven (8%) felt that they stayed too long, and another seven that they did not stay long enough. Very few of the patients (only nine) had had visitors who had been asked to leave; eight of these had been asked by a member of the nursing staff. One visitor had been asked to leave because of a breach of the rules, and two because they had come at the wrong time. The reason for the other five requests was not given.

Only a small number felt that there were too many visitors on the ward in general; the majority (81%) did not think so. Four people said they found too many visitors on the ward tiring, and one felt that the ward was too crowded.

However, slightly more (14 people) felt they had had too many visitors on some occasion. Eight of these said that they had too many at a weekend, one said she had too many visitors every day, and one that she had too many the day after delivery. A similar number (15) felt that *another* patient had had too many visitors at some time, and again a weekend was specified by six. We can see that 59 (68%) of the patients had three or more visitors on some occasion – a number exceeding what is permitted by the rules. However, only fifteen patients (17%) thought their *own* highest number was too many – and the highest number for these patients varied from three to over nine. A similar picture emerges when patients were asked to specify the highest number of visitors another patient had received and to say if they thought this number too many. Again there was evidence that a majority of patients had on some occasion had a number of visitors that exceeded what was allowed, but that this was not seen as 'too many'. There was no evidence of a difference between maternity and gynaecology wards in terms of numbers visiting or problems with visiting.

In general, the patients liked having visitors. Eighteen (20%) found other people's visitors a nuisance, and 15 (17%) had found their own a nuisance. As indicated above, the main reasons given were noise, children becoming unruly, the ward becoming too crowded and finding visitors tiring. However, a large majority found neither their own nor other people's visitors a nuisance, and there was no strong demand for rule enforcement to prevent the perceived problems.

The nurses

General characteristics   All the nurses on the maternity and gynaecological wards were sent questionnaires which they were asked to complete and return to the researchers at the Polytechnic. The response rate was low: 17 completed questionnaires (39.7% of the possible total) were received from nurses working on the maternity wards, and 6 (30%) from those working on gynaecological wards. The majority of those who responded were Registered Nurses or Midwives, and none of the Sisters completed a questionnaire. The response was lower from the gynaecological wards (even allowing for the differences in numbers of nursing staff). This may reflect the fact that it was the maternity nurses who had expressed concern over visiting regulations. The vast majority of the nurses who completed the questionnaire had worked on their current ward for more than one year (17); four had worked there for between six months and a year, and two for less than six months.

Visiting rules   Five of the nurses on the gynaecological wards thought that the existing rules on visiting were satisfactory, but one felt they were unsatisfactory. This nurse and one other thought that the rules were too laxly enforced. Similarly, a majority of the maternity nurses felt that the existing rules were on the whole satisfactory:

It is better not to have visiting during the mornings due to the fact that the ward is generally busier and also the mums need time on their own to learn to care for and get to know their babies. We allow an hour in the evenings for husbands to be alone with their wives and babies.

(Midwife, Ward 21)

I think that the rules are quite satisfactory, if however they are not abused. I agree with patients' own children only allowed to visit because children get bored and start running around which is dangerous because if an emergency occurs they get in the way. Also, visitors not using the smoking room because ours is too small and with a couple of people in the room the air is thick, unfortunately some of the visitors don't abide by the rules.

(Nursing Auxiliary, Ward 9)

It is very nice for husbands to have free visiting, but 2.00 p.m. to 8.00 p.m. is a long time for others.

(Midwife, Ward 11)

Five, however, thought the existing rules on visiting unsatisfactory. One nurse summed up the points made by this group well:

There is often a constant flow of visitors for one or more patients all afternoon. Consequently the patient visited, as well as the others in the room, gets no respite or rest and becomes overtired (often without understanding the reason).

Visitors do not take any notice of the rules either, bringing children in and having half a dozen or so around the bed at once. The midwife is considered the 'big bad wolf' when she tries to enforce the rules and no one appreciates that it is for the protection of the mother and her baby.

It is difficult to carry out care in the post-natal wards when there is a constant stream of visitors for five-and-a-half hours. The mothers may also be reluctant to send visitors away at feed times or if they feel tired or inundated with so many people – they do not want to appear rude or ungrateful. The baby is also over-handled – being passed from one visitor to the next and so becoming overtired and irritable and unsettled leading to a tired, frustrated mother, who often doesn't understand why her baby is 'unsettled'.

She also added, however, that:

Visiting times make things difficult for husbands who work during these times – flexibility is important in these cases.

Eight of the maternity nurses thought that the existing rules were too laxly enforced, and eight that they were administered about right; one person did not respond to this question. One commented that

The midwife on duty is responsible for enforcing the rules and is often too busy to do this effectively, plus the fact that she is often ignored when she does attempt to enforce them.

(Midwife, Ward 10)

Visiting problems and numbers of visitors   All the gynaecological nurses said that there had been occasions when they thought that a patient had had too many visitors – three within the last two weeks and two over two weeks ago but within the last month. Four was the smallest number of visitors and nine the most referred to on these occasions. All the nurses gave as a reason for the number of visitors being too many that it tired the patient excessively but some also talked about inconvenience to other patients or problems created for the nurses. As far as child visitors were concerned, two could not remember a visitor having an excessive number of them, but four could. The occasion had been within the last two weeks in two cases, more than two weeks but less than a month in one, and over a month but within the last year in the final case. The number of children seen as excessive ranged from one to four.

Five of the gynaecology nurses remembered an occasion when they felt that a patient's visitor stayed too long. In three cases this was within the last two weeks, and in two cases between a month and a year ago. The main reason given, again, was that it tired the patient excessively. In one case the patient was thought to be too ill, and in another it was thought to have caused a nuisance to other patients.

However, only one of the gynaecology nurses had ever received a complaint from a patient with regard to the visiting rules, and one a complaint from a visitor – both arguing that the rules were too strict. Five of the gynaecology nurses had had to request visitors to comply with the rules, and three had had to speak to visitors about their conduct on the ward.

Like the gynaecology nurses, all the maternity nurses who worked days (one respondent worked nights) could recall an occasion when they felt that a patient had had too many visitors. Only four could not recall such an occasion within the last year. The number of visitors thought excessive varied from three to twelve. The majority gave as one of their reasons that the number of visitors present tired the patient excessively, but again, inconvenience to other patients and/or problems created for the nurses were also mentioned by some.

One of the nurses, commenting on her reasons for thinking that eight visitors (including two children) was too many, wrote

My objection in this case arose as a patient was post-caesarian section, which included complications during the operation. I suggested to her husband in the morning, after his wife's return to the ward, to advise his family to leave visiting until later in the afternoon. Despite this the family, anxious to see the new baby, arrived within two hours of the operation. The patient was sleeping but they woke her up to let her know they had arrived. The two children belonged to the patient's sister and were left to run unsupervised around the ward until I intervened.

(Midwife, Ward 10)

Four of the maternity nurses could not remember an occasion when they thought that a patient had an excessive number of child visitors. Of the rest, six could recall an occasion within the last two weeks and six an occasion longer than two weeks ago but less than a year. The numbers mentioned as being excessive ranged from two to five. Again, the main reason given was that the patient was tired excessively; a number made the point that children were left unsupervised and three pointed out that the children in question were not the patient's own.

> The children are often allowed to run up and down the corridors unchecked by their parents and so disturb other patients. The children may also be prone to accident if not watched by their parents, as staff do not have time to watch that they do not get up to mischief or fall over, etc.
>
> (Midwife, Ward 10)

Twelve of the maternity nurses could recall an occasion when they felt a patient's visitors had stayed too long. Six of these occasions were in the last two weeks, and only one over a year ago. Again, the main reason given was that the length of the visit tired the patient excessively; additionally, six said that the length of visit exceeded what was allowed by the rules, and inconvenience to other patients, problems for nurses and the fact that the children were not supervised were also reported.

Ten of the nurses recalled having received a complaint about the visiting rules from a patient, three of these being within the last two weeks. Four of the complaints were related to what was seen as too restricted visiting hours. The remainder were concerned that they or another patient had had too many visitors, or visitors that had stayed too long or were disruptive:

> Too many visitors during the day. Feeling tired and tearful at the end of the day.
>
> (Midwife, Ward 11)

> Patients felt tired as visitors came all afternoon and evening with no respite. She would have liked a bath but didn't like to ask visitors to leave and felt she had to rush her supper because all her visitors were there.
>
> (Midwife, Ward 11)

> Neighbouring patients' visitors were noisy and disturbing, giving no consideration to other patients in the room.
>
> (Midwife, Ward 10)

> Patient complained whilst I was writing answers that all had had too many visitors over a period and all had stayed too long!
>
> (Midwife, Ward 10)

Only seven of the maternity nurses had received a complaint from a visitor regarding the visiting rules. One of these was that the rules were being broken by visitors to his/her relative and that this was upsetting the patient. The remainder all concerned the restrictions of the rules: one objected to not being allowed to smoke on the ward and the remainder to the hours permitted (one objecting because visiting finished at 7.30 p.m. and not 8.00 p.m. as on other wards).

All but one of the maternity nurses had had to ask visitors to comply with the rules on visiting, eleven of them within the last two weeks. The main reason given for having to speak to visitors was that there were too many – seven respondents mentioned this. Five nurses spoke to visitors because they had come outside normal visiting hours or had stayed on after visiting had finished, thus preventing the patient getting sufficient rest, or in three cases coming in the morning, preventing nurses carrying out nursing procedures. Three nurses said that the patient was too unwell to cope with the number of visitors, two said that child visitors were causing problems, and one that the visitors were taking the baby out of an incubator. (Note that the numbers add up to more than 100 per cent of the respondents because some respondents gave more than one reason.) Twelve nurses had had to talk to visitors about their behaviour on the ward. All the reported incidents, with the exception of one, had occurred in the last year (and four within the last two weeks). On six occasions this had been because the visitors were noisy and in some cases using bad language (two nurses saying that the people concerned were drunk). Three parents had been asked to control their children, two groups of visitors not to handle the baby too much, and one partner not to lie on the patient's bed.

Perceptions of patient preference   Eight of the nurses thought that the patients liked the existing visiting arrangements. One said that patients would prefer a shorter visiting period. Seven thought that patients would like a break between afternoon and evening visiting, but one of these and one other thought that patients would like visiting time to start an hour earlier in the afternoon and four thought they would like open visiting during the day. Finally, one thought that patients' views on visiting would depend on how well or unwell they felt.

Fifteen of the nurses said that patients like being visited frequently. Three said that patients would prefer two separate visiting periods, afternoon and evening, and to be visited in both. One further nurse qualified her answer by saying that patients would prefer not to have visits in the morning or during meal-times and not to have all the visitors at once. One made a distinction between what she thought ante-natal and post-natal patients would like:

> Ante-natally, as often as possible to relieve the boredom. Post-natally – quite often as long as it fitted around caring for and feeding the baby and as long as they got enough rest.

With respect to the hours visitors would like, fifteen thought that they would like open visiting, while seven said they thought that visitors liked the present hours. Two gave answers which indicated that they thought patients would prefer fewer visits.

Nurses' own preferences for visiting   Finally, the nurses were asked questions about how they thought visiting ought to be organized. Nine said that from the point of view of the nursing staff the visiting hours should stay as at present. Eight of the nurses on maternity wards wanted a break between afternoon and evening visiting. One wanted visiting restricted to afternoons only and another to the period from 4.00 p.m. to 8.00 p.m. Two wanted an extended period of afternoon/evening visiting, and two said that visiting should be allowed all day. However, eleven of the nurses thought that visiting should be different from the point of view of the patient. Four who had said that visiting should be restricted to afternoon/evening from the point of view of nurses said that from the patients' point of view visiting should be open. A further two thought that visiting hours would be longer if patients' views were consulted than if the nurses were. Two thought that patients would like a longer break between afternoon and evening visiting than was necessary from a nurse's point of view. Nevertheless a slight majority (14) thought that patients' and nurses' points of view were essentially the same.

Nine of the nurses agreed with the present rules on numbers of visitors – two at any one time; a further four said the number should be restricted to two or three. Six nurses thought the number should be limited to three, three to four, and one said it depended on the condition of the patient. However, thirteen nurses thought there should be no restriction on the number of visitors allowed during the course of the day. The other ten all thought the total number permitted during the day should be restricted. Six thought that six visitors should be the maximum number allowed, two that visitors should be restricted to four a day, one to three a day, and one to not more than ten.

All the nurses thought that a patient's own children should be allowed to visit her, although one felt that babies and very young children should not be allowed. However, only seven thought that children other than the patients' own should be allowed, and two of them qualified their answers – one saying only grandchildren and the other only the children of close relatives or friends. Seven of the nurses thought that adult visiting should be restricted to close relatives; five of them worked on the maternity wards and two on the gynaecological wards.

Finally, four of the nurses thought that the rules on visiting should be the same throughout the hospital. The rest thought they should vary according to the needs of the staff and patients on particular wards – for example, two specifically mentioned that visiting should be open on children's wards for parents, and another referred to the specific needs of the maternity unit. The quoted passages below sum up to these views:

> There should be more restriction on post-natal wards to allow mothers to adjust to motherhood and caring for and learning to know their new babies. As well as rest to avoid extreme fatigue, ante-natal patients need visitors to dispel boredom. Labour ward patients should only have the people they want with them for as long as they like.
>
> (Midwife, Ward 10)

Patients are not ill on maternity on the whole, so can cope with more visitors at a time (four instead of two). Maternity in particular needs a 'partners only' time. Patients in maternity usually only stay a short time (three to four days), so visiting could be limited to close relatives, whereas in other areas, with patients staying in longer, they probably need a variety of visitors.

There is concern, then, among the nurses about the existing arrangements. While a majority seem relatively satisfied, there is a substantial minority who express concern. Most of the nurses can remember recent occasions when visitors have broken the visiting rules, and a substantial minority's responses indicate that they would like to see the rules more strictly enforced. There is, however, some recognition that patients would not like visiting to be more restricted, and some realization that there may be a disjunction between what the nurses would find most suitable as visiting arrangements and what the patients would want.

Discussion and conclusions

The survey seems to indicate that, on the whole, patients and visitors are satisfied with the visiting arrangements as they are. When we say 'arrangements as they are', we mean literally just that: we are including the informal variations of the formal rules. The actual practices 'on the ground' are rather different from either the PCHC's intention of having no time-limited access between 2.00 p.m. and 8.00 p.m., and the rules governing numbers which are stated in notices and communications to incoming patients. Such variations should be no cause for anxiety: all large organizations have this behavioural pattern, and a concern for administrative tidiness or strict exercise of authority should not be allowed to obscure the reality that the human beings most affected – patients, nurses and visitors – have evolved a compromise which the research shows to be working quite well.

However, it is also clear that the majority of patients and visitors want patients to be allowed to have more visitors at a time than are allowed by the present rules. The majority of patients do not think they have ever had too many visitors at once, nor that another patient on their ward has had too many. A small number of patients have been disturbed by too many visitors, generally because they could not cope, they felt too tired or children were a nuisance, but this was a relatively minor problem.

We suggest that these difficulties could be tackled in three simple ways. First, consideration should be given to how far the principle of open visiting could be sacrificed to allow a meal break for maternity unit patients. Normally (but with the current sensible flexibility) there would be no visitors at this time. Second, the rules should be slightly modified, to recognize more fully the need for partners to visit at varying times, and to allow three, not two, as the maximum number of visitors per patient. These rules would then be more carefully enforced. Thus we see both a tightening and a liberation of the rules over visiting.

Third, it is important to recognize that such changes require nurses and visitors to modify their present behaviour. The nurses are the people 'at the sharp end' who would have to enforce the rules. They would need to be helped, by *training*, to see the new pattern of control as a legitimate professional activity. Intervention with visitors requires advanced interpersonal skills in order to retain the current patient/visitor goodwill while at the same time achieving the goals of some limiting of access. There is little possibility of successful change without the introduction of a specific, albeit short, programme of training. The visitors in turn can be helped to see what behaviour is appropriate during visits. Some thought could be given to modifying the briefing which patients and partners receive, and to the information which could be given to every visitor. For example, there are still visitors who have little idea of how long a visit should last. Some seem to think open visiting is a requirement to spend from 2.00 p.m. to 8.00 p.m. with the patient!

It should also be pointed out that most of the problems which the research has identified are not unique to either a formal or informal version of open visiting. They are to be found to some degree in *all* systems of hospital visiting. While it is true that highly restrictive hours, or rigidly enforced control of numbers, may reduce the risk of over-tiring patients and disrupting hospital routines, they equally cause other problems particularly for the patients and visitors but additionally for the nurses who have to enforce such systems. No system is without its costs.

How do women and men in nursing perceive each other?

George Choon and Suzanne Skevington

Stereotyping the sexes

Repeatedly, studies have shown that people have different expectations about the two sexes and their behaviour. Within any culture there is a high degree of consensus between people about the nature of these differences. For example, Williams *et al.* (1975) asked students to decide which of 300 adjectives were associated with men or women. They were able to classify 90% of these items, and had 75% agreement about which were which. Women were said to be affectionate, appreciative, gentle, charming, weak, prudish, fussy, and nagging for instance; while men were seen as adventurous, realistic, independent, rational, boastful, loud, and daring, among other things. Rosencrantz and colleagues (1968) in a similar experiment, found that when they asked about which characteristics were socially desirable, masculine characteristics were seen as much more socially desirable than feminine ones. In other words, women were less highly valued than men on a wide variety of dimensions.

Only a brief review of the many studies in this area can be set out here (see Fransella and Frost, 1977, for an extended appraisal) but Reece (1964) indicates that two dimensions are important when the stereotypes of women and men are being measured. The first is *potency*; where men are seen as consistently more powerful, strong, and robust. The second is *social behaviour*, where women are seen as more considerate towards others, and more sensible.

To summarize, there is a strong consensus that men and women are different, and that they differ according to age, religion, marital status, and educational level. In addition, characteristics ascribed to men are valued more positively than those ascribed to women. Finally, not only are these stereotypes acknowledged by both women and men, but they are absorbed into the self-concepts which men and women hold about themselves (Broverman *et al.*, 1972). More recently, Bem (1981) has looked more closely at people's views of their gender. Simplifying a complex argument, she says that these perceptions of our masculinity or femininity act as a filter through which all events in our world are viewed, as this is called our *gender schema*. . . .

Who is 'Fred' Nightingale?

While people have become more aware of sex discrimination as a result of the legislation of the last two decades, in this climate of change, is there room for 'Fred' Nightingale within the nursing profession?

The material in the previous section suggests that there is a paradox for men entering the profession. Nursing is a caring profession which attracts a majority of women, largely because society demands that, as women, they should be brought up to be caring and warm among other things. Men attracted to nursing, for whatever reason, have to show themselves to be caring also, and this is the reverse of the traditional stereotype of a masculine man. Not only do they have to face being a statistical minority in a world of women, but more importantly they are likely to have their maleness questioned, and to find themselves less socially desirable by taking on the less valued characteristics normally attributed to the female sex. Needless to say, men entering nursing face similar problems to women who have tried to enter areas of work traditionally allocated to men, namely engineering, mining, and the priesthood.

Siegal (1977) noted that interest in possible future occupations was sex-linked as early as in primary school children. She found 70% of the girls preferred either nursing or teaching, while the boys showed more diverse vocational preferences in choosing 20 different occupations. In an American nationwide study, Prediger *et al.* (1974) reported that over 50% of the girls in secondary education selected vocational occupations, namely education and social services, nursing, human care, and clerical-secretarial work. Only 7% of the boys selected these occupations, with the rest choosing occupations in engineering, natural sciences, business management, or in other technologies and trades. Similarly Shinar (1975) demonstrated sex stereotypes of occupation in college students, and these were consistently sex-linked. Other studies (e.g. Knudsen, 1969) showed that women had been led to anticipate and prepare for occupations consistent with traditional divisions of labour.

Albrecht (1976) sought to differentiate the sex-role stereotyping of 15 different occupations. Looking more specifically at work in the Health Service, he found that 67% of his respondents agreed that medicine was equally suitable for men as women, 27% agreed that it was more suitable for men than women, but only 1% that it was more suitable for women than men. On the other hand, nursing was regarded as equally suitable for both women and men by only 36%, more suitable for women than men by 55%, but more suitable for men than women by only 1%. So it seems reasonable to conclude that sex-role stereotyping is quite powerful in influencing occupational choice here. Fred Nightingale would seem to be a person who is able to avoid or resist the stereotyping of traditional sex roles.

However, the picture is clouded by more complexities. Men in the Health Service tend not to be in subordinate positions. The image of male–female relationships tends to be one of the male doctor and the female nurse. Leeson and Gray (1978) have suggested that the distribution of power and earnings between the sexes in the Health Service mirrors not only the position of men and women in society as a whole, but more specifically the roles of the sexes inside the family, and this view is supported by Webb (1982) in *Nursing Mirror*. Within nurses as a group, women have tended to see themselves as of higher status than male nurses, so the men entering nursing tend to find themselves at the bottom of the hierarchy within a low status job.

How have they coped with this? In interview male nurses frequently concede that having entered nursing, they are likely to be promoted quickly into positions of seniority, and the statistics bear this out. In 1971, on average, there were seven women for every man in post. However, looking at the senior posts of chief and principal nursing officer and charge nurse, the proportion of women to men was only three to one. The proportion of women to men increases as the ranks are descended so that at the bottom of the hierarchy there were eleven women pupil nurses for each man in training. It is clear that men are overrepresented at senior level and underrepresented at junior level when compared with the average number in this population. Parallels can be drawn with other areas of women's work, such as catering and hairdressing, where men are also promoted to positions of power and responsibility which far exceed their expected representation in the population. This indicates that there is a bias favouring the promotion of men in preference to women.

So why does this occur? There are no simple answers, but one recent piece of research suggests that women and men learn different sets of beliefs during their childhood and adolescence. This socialization encourages the development of differences between the sexes in the way they view success and failure, and more particularly their perceptions of the *causes* of those successes and failures. Attributional theory is about the study of causation, and has been applied to the area of gender differences by Dweck and Licht (1980). Young men, they say, use a number of coping strategies to shrug off failure, which protect them from believing that failure is anything to do with their lack of ability. Instead of blaming themselves, they tend to blame others or factors beyond their control for failure. Young women on the other hand, learn to believe that failure is directly due to their own personal lack of ability, and as a result of realizing their limitations, failure tends to deter them from trying to succeed again much more than their male counterparts. It seems that it is not a *real* lack of ability, but the *perception* that they lack it, which reduces their potential to achieve, and this could be an important psychological reason why they do not put themselves forward for promotion and are seen to lack ambition both in nursing and elsewhere. So while there are substantial psychological deterrents to entering nurse training, once embarked upon a career in nursing, Fred Nightingale is in an advantageous position both structurally and psychologically to move quickly into areas of power and prestige.

The stereotypes of nurses

What do nurses think about their own characteristics, the characteristics of opposite sex nurses, and of different types of nurses? Hoffman (1970) found that general nurses scored higher than the normal population on such traits as nurturance, order desirability, and harm-avoidance, but fell below the average for aggression, autonomy, change, and dominance. Gynther and Gertz (1962) found general nurses scored higher on endurance, orderliness, and deference, but lower on exhibition and achievement.

Reich and Geller (1977) reported that psychiatric nurses described themselves as serious, cautious, methodical, cooperative, and able to relate well with others. They also found that nurses rejected self-concepts such as timid and submissive, and they preferred to think of themselves as aggressive, assertive, self-confident and independent. They concluded that nurses working in a psychiatric field have a strong identification with many of the values of psychiatry, namely self-control, self-assertion and achievement. This may account for the differences in self-image between the psychiatric nurses and the general nursing group.

Caine and Small (1969) obtained marked differences in attitudes and interests between nurses in general hospitals and those working in psychiatric hospitals. Reavley and Wilson (1972) also concluded that there were marked differences between male and female nurses on three factors of the Cattell 16 Personality Factors Test, but this difference was seen only on one of these dimensions after less than a year in training, suggesting that the group was very homogeneous. These studies are important in showing how particular personality predispositions tend to be associated with different types of nurses and nursing. Reavley and Wilson's finding that perceived differences between men and women nurses are dissipated during training and with contact, is particularly important in illustrating the arbitrariness of the divisions created by sex-role stereotypes.

It seems possible that men entering a women's world to work may have a different view of the other sex than those who choose to enter traditional areas of men's work. The Briggs Report (1972) admits that for many men, nursing is a second choice, but they do see it as a 'positive shift to a more worthwhile job'. It is an interesting area of study because, since the passing of the Sex Discrimination Act 1975 we need to know more about the psychological effects of entry into other-sex jobs of people who belong to a minority category. In the main study reported here we have looked at how nurses see themselves, and the other group, and also how nurses of one sex believe that those of the other sex see them. The latter is described as a *metaperspective* by Laing *et al.* (1966).

The study of nurses' stereotypes

Psychiatric nurses were chosen for study because men form a large minority group in the population, and any stereotypes formed would have been based on a certain amount of information gained from personal contact, unlike general hospital populations or midwifery, where male nurses working on the wards are uncommon or non-existent. It is worth noting, however, that as psychiatry is not seen as women's work like general nursing, so the beliefs may differ from those of the general population of male nurses portrayed by earlier studies. Burns (1977) developed the Semantic Differential Questionnaire (BSDQ) to investigate men's and women's perceptions of their own and the other sex. Using a sample of Open University adult students, he showed that men and women still saw themselves, and were being perceived by members of the other sex, in the traditional sex-role stereotypes. Men were stereotyped by women as strong, active, aggressive, dominant, and emotionally in control. Women perceived themselves, and were viewed by men, as emotionally labile, dependent, passive, weak, conservative, kind, affectionate, and warm. Burns concluded that his semantic differential questionnaire enabled each sex to differentiate between its psychological characteristics and those of the other sex, and each sex agreed to a fair degree on the characteristics given to itself by the other sex.

The semantic differential is a useful tool for measuring opposite concepts, e.g. dominant versus submissive, cooperative versus competitive. Using the seven points between the two poles the respondent shows how much and how little of the two characteristics he or she thinks he or she possesses. Twenty-one scales of this type were given to 99 psychiatric nurses (28 men and 71 women), and were used to find out what nurses thought about their own sex group and the other sex group, as well as what they thought the other group thought about them (metaperspective). The age of the nurses was 17 to 42 (average 20.6 years) (see Table 7.1).

Looking at those characteristics in this study which were marked a substantial distance (1.5 units) away from the midpoint of the scale (the midpoint was 4 on a scale from one to seven) it was found that women nurses perceived themselves as kind, happy, and tending to show affection; and men saw themselves as never crying. In both cases a mixture of masculine and feminine stereotypes was also present. For example, active and intelligent were included in women's perceptions of themselves, while men saw themselves as cooperative, expressing anger verbally and cautious. However, more traditional stereotypes emerged when nurses gave ratings of the opposite sex. Men see women as more cautious, having unpredictable moods, and crying easily, while women see men as independent and never crying.

This traditional stereotype seems to become even more extreme when the metaperspective results are examined. Men think women see men as dominant, aggressive, and never crying, in other words an image which conflicts with their image of themselves; while women think that men see women as kind, warm, crying easily, tending to show affection and taking things personally – a stereotype which only partly reflects the image the group holds of itself. Comparisons were made between these perceptions using statistical tests (t-tests) to see if there were any differences between the ways in which people perceive each other, and the way they believe that others perceive them.

Table 7.1   The semantic differential
Instructions
Below you will find a *concept* to be judged, and beneath it a set of scales. You are to rate the *concept* of each of the 21 scales on a 7 point basis. The direction towards which you put a *cross* depends upon which of the two ends of each scale seem most characteristic of your judgement.

Your perception of the male[1] nurse

1. Dominant	Submissive
2. Cooperative	Competitive
3. Aggressive	Peaceful
4. Kind	Unkind
5. Independent	Dependent
6. Weak	Powerful
7. Cold	Warm
8. Conformist	Non-comformist
9. Active	Passive
10. Cautious	Reckless
11. Logical	Intuitive
12. Conservative	Radical
13. Stable	Neurotic
14. Stupid	Intelligent
15. Sees things objectively	Takes things personally
16. Uncreative	Creative
17. Predictable moods	Unpredictable moods
18. Expresses anger verbally	Expresses anger physically
19. Never cries	Cries easily
20. Tends to show affection	Does not show affection
21. Happy	Sad

[1] In other versions, the words 'female', 'female's view of the male nurse', or 'male nurse's view of the female nurse', were substituted.

What are the perceived characteristics of nurses regardless of sex? Both female and male nurses alike see their groups as kind, active, cautious, stable, intelligent, creative, and happy, although they do not acknowledge that the other sex group has all these qualities too, so there is a mismatch of perceptions. When male nurses compare the sexes they see women as predominantly weak, unstable, cautious, likely to take things personally, to have unpredictable moods, and to cry easily. When female nurses compare the sexes they see men as more competitive, aggressive, unkind, powerful, cold, nonconformist, reckless, radical, likely to see things objectively, and less likely to show affection or cry, and in a minor way they do acknowledge creativity. So while there is some agreement between the sexes about the qualities present among nurses, there is considerable disparity between the way sex groups see themselves and the way they perceive the other sex group. Male nurses also see men in nursing as cooperative, kind, cautious, logical, creative and able to express anger verbally – these characteristics are traditionally feminine ones.

Reich and Geller (1977) reported that psychiatric nurses described themselves as cautious, methodical, cooperative, and able to relate well to others, and the present findings tend to be in agreement with these results. But male nurses did not see themselves as aggressive and independent; they were seen more in line with Hoffman's (1970) results of nurturance and harm-avoidance. Men working in female-dominated occupations probably find these sex-role stereotypes desirable and effective in the execution of their work.

Turning now to the beliefs nurses held about the other sex-group's perceptions of them. Here there was agreement with traditional sex-role stereotyping from both male and female nurses. Male nurses believed female nurses would stereotype male nurses as dominant, aggressive and happy. Female nurses believed male nurses would stereotype women nurses as kind, weak, warm, conformist, cautious, conservative, taking things personally, tending to show affection, having unpredictable moods, crying easily and happy. The nurses' understanding of the other sex nurses' views was sex-typed, producing extreme stereotypes of both male and female nurses. This differed to a large extent from their actual self-perceptions. . . .

Men entering nursing do see themselves as having a number of so-called feminine characteristics, but these aspects of their self-image seem to be denied by some female nurses. There are two main interpretations of these results. Firstly, it could be that the male nurses' self-image is for 'publicity' purposes, and that they do not behave in accordance with their proclaimed beliefs about themselves, or alternatively it is possible that women nurses do not want to see the 'feminine' side of their male colleagues for a whole host of defensive reasons.

Both male and female nurses rated nurses of their own sex higher on opposite sex items. It would seem that women nurses in this female-dominated profession found the male characteristics less desirable, whereas male nurses found the female characteristics more desirable so as, presumably, to enable them to work better with women. This may be due, of course, to adaptability as more male nurses become attracted to the profession. It is not possible to conclude whether men entering nursing were selected because they had these qualities, or whether they developed these qualities during training.

The nurses also revealed many significantly different items between their actual perceptions and their beliefs of the other sex nurses' views of the opposite sex nurse. These items tended to reflect traditional sex-role stereotypes and were extreme for either sex nurses. A belief seems to exist that nurses of one sex will stereotype the opposite sex nurse in a highly traditional way. This belief may result in a conflict arising from misconceptions about what the opposite sex nurses think of them. As such, these findings appear to have considerable implications for the training and selection of male and female nurses.

Conclusion

The present findings indicate that in terms of self-perceptions, perceptions of opposite sex, and beliefs of opposite sex perceptions, there is a consistent and highly significant pattern of differences between male and female nurses, which might be attributable to sex-role stereotyping. Generally, the professional qualities popularly stereotyped as feminine, i.e. kind, warm, cautious, affectionate, are highly rated by both female and male nurses in their self-perceptions. However, female nurses do not perceive male nurses to possess these qualities and the perpetuation of such sex-role stereotypes in selection, training, and professional practice may be damaging in preventing men from entering the profession, although it seems clear from the statistics that they are given highly preferential treatment once trained, in a way which must make the talented women in nursing feel resentful and threatened, and even more determined to maintain nursing as women's work.

References

Albrecht, S. L. (1976). Social class and sex-stereotyping of occupations. *Journal of Vocational Behaviour*, 9(3), 321–328.

Bem, S. L. (1981). Gender schema theory: a cognitive account of sex typing. *Psychological Review*, 88, 354–364.

Briggs, A. (1972). *Report of the Committee on Nursing*. Cmnd 5115. HMSO, London.

Broverman, I. K., Vogel, S. R., Broverman, D. M., Clarkson, F. E. and Rosenkrantz, P. S. (1972). Sex-role stereotypes: a current appraisal. *Journal of Social Issues*, 28, 59–78.

Burns, R. B. (1977). Male and female perceptions of their own and other sex. *British Journal of Social and Clinical Psychology*, 16(3), 213–200.

Caine, T. M. and Small, D. J. (1969). *The Treatment of Mental Illness*. University of London Press, London.

Dweck, C. S. and Licht, B. G. (1980). 'Learned helplessness and intellectual achievement,' in *Human Helplessness: theory and applications*. (eds J. Garber and M. E. P. Seligman). pp.197–222. Academic Press, London.

Fransella, F. and Frost, K. (1977). *On Being a Woman*. Tavistock, London.

Gynther, M. D. and Gertz, B. (1962). Personality characteristics of student nurses in South Carolina. *Journal of Psychology*, 56, 277–284.

Hoffman, H. (1970). Note on the personality traits of student nurses. *Psychological Reports*, 27, 1004.

Knudsen, D. D. (1969). The declining status of women: Popular myths and the failure of functionalist thought. *Social Forces*, 48, 183–193.

Laing, R. D., Phillipson, H. and Lee, A. R. (1966). *Interpersonal Perception*. Tavistock, London.

Leeson, J. and Gray, J. (1978). *Women and Medicine*. Tavistock, London.

Prediger, D. J., Roth, J. D. and Noeth, R. J. (1974). Career development of youth: A nationwide study. *Personnel and Guidance Journal*, 53, 97–104.

Reavley, W. and Wilson, L. J. (1972). Personality structure of general and psychiatric student nurses: a comparison. *International Journal of Nursing Studies*, 9, 225–234.

Reece, M. M. (1964). Masculinity and femininity: a factor analytic study. *Psychological Reports*, 14, 123–139.

Reich, S. and Geller, A. (1977). The self-image of nurses employed in a psychiatric hospital. *Perspectives in Psychiatric Care*, 15(3), 126–128.

Shinar, E. H. (1975). Sexual stereotypes of occupations. *Journal of Vocational Behaviour*, 7, 99–111.

Siegal, C. L. E. (1977). Sex differences in the occupational choices of second graders. *Journal of Vocational Behaviour*, 3, 15–19.

Webb, C. (1982). The men wear the trousers, *Nursing Mirror*, 154(2), 29–31.

Williams, J. E., Bennett, S. M. and Best, D. L. (1975). Awareness and expression of sex stereotypes in young children. *Developmental Psychology*, 11(5), 635–642.

≡ Section C ≡

Controlled trials and comparisons

Introduction

In this final section we look at examples of the most internally structured kind of research design – experiments and other designs which attempt to follow the same logic as experiments. The *experiment* (or *controlled trial*) expresses a simple logic: that if you manipulate one variable and observe that another one changes, and you can show that there is no other plausible explanation for the observed change except for the manipulation you introduced, then you may argue that your manipulation caused the change. In the simplest and clearest design there would be two identical groups of people, one of whom received a treatment while the other did not. To the extent that the groups *are* identical, and underwent precisely the same experiences during the research except for the presence or absence of the treatment, we may say that any observed effect is *caused* by the treatment. Verona Gordon's contribution in this section (Chapter 8) describes an experiment of this kind, on the treatment of depression in women. There are other kinds of design, involving multiple comparison or changes over time in the treatment of the same person or people, see for example Sapsford and Abbott (1992) for details. Their underlying principles are the same, however – manipulation of an independent variable to produce changes in a dependent variable, while all extraneous influences (possible alternative explanations) are controlled.

This kind of 'scientific' research has always been popular among 'applied' researchers – researchers into policy or practice – because it impresses managers, administrators and policy-makers. It has 'the authority of science' behind it and appears to deal in 'hard facts' rather than 'subjective opinions'. It does indeed have many strengths, and it is the proper way to proceed where the topic under investigation is well understood and what is at stake is the testing of unambiguous hypotheses. Its power is sometimes overrated, however. As we said earlier, it is good for testing theory, but not good for generating theory, because it is inevitably cast in terms of preconceived concepts and is not open to discovery. It is also *reductionist* – it identifies 'variables' for manipulation and/or measurement – and often has difficulty relating these back to the lives and social worlds of those under investigation and the social structures within which they operate. Policy-makers have been 'educated' by the research which has been presented to them, over the years, and more 'qualitative' work is now often equally acceptable to them. Nonetheless this kind of controlled comparison remains a strong set of techniques and useful for the applied researcher.

Many classic experiments of social psychology take place in the laboratory, under controlled conditions, and are therefore open to attack on the grounds that the situation is totally unnatural – what happens in the laboratory might well not happen in ordinary life. Many others escape this criticism by taking place in a real-life setting, and this would include virtually all experimental testing of new treatment procedures and professional practices. If the subjects know that they are a part of an experiment there is an automatic alternative explanation for their behaviour – that they may be behaving as they are in order to comply with the 'rules of experiments'. (This is known as the Hawthorne Effect, after a famous piece of real-life research in which every change made to working conditions in a factory improved productivity – including undoing all the changes and putting things back to how they had been before the study!) It is frequent practice, therefore, to conceal the purpose of the research from the experimental subjects. Many would argue, however, that there is something unethical in manipulating subjects without their knowledge and consent, that it amounts to treating them as objects rather than human beings.

Verona Gordon's experiment, in Chapter 8 in this section, passes muster in this respect – her subjects knew perfectly well what was going on. It is also worth noting that her experiment does no harm to subjects and puts no-one at risk of harm or distress – something which cannot be said for all. She even avoids the charge very often levelled at controlled trials in therapy or education, that it is immoral to withhold treatment from a control group just for the sake of the experimental design. With limited resources she could handle only a relatively small number of clients in her therapy groups, and she had a large number of applicants, so she did not so much withhold treatment from the control group as capitalize on the fact that she could not deal with everyone who applied. Thus we may put her study forward as a good example of this kind of research. However, we should note that that the ethical problems of experimentation are considerable; experimental designs give rise to even more misgivings and questions that need answering than other kinds of research.

Often true experiments are impossible even in principle. In the second contribution in this section (Chapter 9), for example, Dingwall and Fox compare the reactions of social workers and health visitors to a standard stimulus. The independent variable is 'being a social worker' versus 'being a health visitor', and there is no way that this difference can be under the control of the researcher. Nonetheless the comparison proceeds *quasi*-experimentally, *as if* this were a true experiment, and causal conclusions are drawn about the differences in response between the two kinds of professional. The argument is obviously weak: social workers and health visitors may differ from each other on a whole range of characteristics (class, education, background, personality, professional experience, professional socialization), and we will not know what is interesting about any significant difference without a fair amount of further study. (Correlation does not prove causation: differences between the two groups could be due to one or more of the variables put forward above, rather than to the difference in immediate job.) Choon and Skevington's chapter in the last section, similarly, was a quasi-experimental comparison because the independent variable is gender, and this is not under the control of the researcher. Gender might signify biological differences, or differences in socialization, or differences in social experience as a 'stimulus-object', or differences in social expectation, or any of a whole range of other gender differences or an interaction between any or all of these. The quasi-experimental comparison is logically weaker than the true experiment, and more research may be needed before we can put a sensible interpretation on the results.

Frequently quasi-experimental comparison is used where the true experiment is not impossible in principle, but totally unethical in practice. In Chapter 10, Abbott *et al.* illustrate this kind of research. It would not be impossible in principle to allocate some people to materially deprived families and others to materially advantaged ones – it is not beyond the powers of an extremely unethical adoption agency. In practice, however, in researching this kind of topic one has to look at what exists, rather than manipulating conditions, and this is what the Abbott *et al.* chapter does (following a substantial tradition of similar research). It explores the correlation between the material deprivation of areas and their health status – a different analytic technique from that of Dingwall and Fox or Choon and Skevington, but following the same logic of exploring how an independent variable affects a dependent variable – in this case, how material deprivation affects health status, ward by ward in one Health District.

Another point to note about this chapter is that researchers do not always have to collect their own data. This chapter uses the census and the statistics on birth and death – two major sets of statistics collected and published by governmental agencies. There are many others which can also be useful for answering questions such as those which Abbott *et al.* raise. For a discussion of some of them, and their strengths and drawbacks, see Sapsford and Abbott (1992).

Reference

Sapsford, R. and Abbott, P. (1992). *Research Methods for Nurses and the Caring Professions*. Open University Press, Buckingham.

## 8

Treatment of depressed women by nurses

Verona Gordon

Introduction

Depression ranks as one of the major health problems of women today. Although prominent researchers Weissman and Klerman (1970) reported that twice as many women are depressed as men around the world, few research studies have been published on the development and utilization of treatment approaches to meet the needs of this population. The widespread growth in the number of American females of all ages suffering from depression is alarming (Guttentag and Belle, 1980). Depressed women have increased medical costs due to their repeated visits to physicians for psychosomatic complaints, chemical dependency, unnecessary gynaecological surgery, and their high psychiatric hospitalizations. Women seek counselling; however, there have been few convincing research studies on the effectiveness of traditional psychotherapies (Fiske *et al.*, 1970). Due to the rising high cost of health care, treatment approaches in mental health must be efficacious, safe and cost-effective (Parloff, 1980). Accelerating societal change is having an impact on women. The challenges to traditional values, roles, and expectations are a source of concern to women and generate emotional responses. Depression is one such emotional response that has been found to be a significant problem among women. Prevention of depression among this segment of society requires an understanding of women's perceptions of, and concerns about, their life situations. Women have high potential to learn, strong interest in growing, great influence over their families, and much to give others.

The purpose of this chapter is to provide more information about the phenomenon of depression in women and to describe a nurse group intervention designed by the author to alleviate depression in women . . .

Review of the literature

Forty million Americans suffer from depression today and two-thirds of these people are women (Hirschfield, 1980). Eminent researchers (Dohrenwend, 1973; van Keep and Prill, 1975; Tucker, 1977; Notman, 1979) identified stressors occurring in women's daily lives which stem from personal, family, social, and cultural demands upon them. These result in feelings of frustration, inadequacy, and low self-esteem.

Problems facing women as they age in America include marital conflicts (Cherlin, 1981), divorce (Gordon, 1979), loss of attractiveness (Scarf, 1980), conflicts at work (Powell, 1977; Shields, 1980), career disruptions due to husband's job change (Weissman *et al.*, 1973), hysterectomy surgery (Raphael, 1976; Editorial, 1979; Martin *et al.*, 1980), 'empty-nest' syndrome (Bart, 1971; Radloff 1975), menopause (Neugarten *et al.*, 1963), widowhood (Lopata, 1971), declining physical health (Wittenborn and Buhler, 1979), and care of elderly parents (Stevenson, 1977). These factors may result in feelings of loneliness and isolation (Gordon, 1982). (There is concern in America in respect to woman's influential role in her family and that she has the longest life expectancy, 78 years versus males 70 years, and earns over half of the nation's income).

Psychological explanations

There may be three aetiological explanations for these escalating rates of depression in American women as described by theories of:

1. Lewinsohn's behavioural model,
2. Seligman's learned helplessness model,
3. Beck's cognitive model.

From the behavioural viewpoint depression occurs when a women does not perceive positive reinforcement in her daily life (Lewinsohn *et al.*, 1982). The highest rate of depression in American females occurs between the ages of 25 and 44 years, probably their response to their own high expectations of work, marriage or having children. Belle (1982) found low-income single mothers most vulnerable to depression and that the rate of psychiatric treatment of their children was high. Most women working full-time earn 59 per cent less than male full-time workers for doing the same job (Barrett, 1979). Eighty per cent of all women working in America tend to work in demanding 'service' jobs (factory work, cleaning, clerical, bank tellers, sales) which are low in pay and prestige (National Commission on Working Women, 1979). Women who are employed find social-financial inequality, sex-role stereotyping, and negative prejudice, which result in reduced self-fulfilment and career options (Clayton *et al.*, 1980; Carmen *et al.*, 1981).

Unemployed, married women consistently report frustration with their roles (Neuberry *et al.*, 1979). Housewives have few sources of gratification

(Thurnher, 1976; Radloff and Rae, 1979): their work is relatively invisible and given little value or prestige. The absence of intimate supportive relationships with husband or children increase the risk of depression (Brown *et al.*, 1975; Miller, 1976). The fact that depression is more common among married, divorced or separated women than men is well documented (Radloff, 1975). Gove (1972) reported that the strain of the marriage role is a causal factor of the higher rate of depression among women. The divorce rate in the United States has increased 96 per cent in the last decade and 50 per cent of all future marriages are predicted to end in divorce (*Los Angeles Times*, 1980). The stress of divorce is felt more by women than by men due to women's lack of money, poor living conditions, and lack of job skills (Maykowsky, 1980). Due to present national economy, there are a growing number of women staying in loveless, empty, and abusive marriages (Kaslow, 1982). Pilisuk and Froland (1978) write that depression in women will continue to increase with the high mobility (extended families living thousands of miles apart), small family size, and high divorce rates.

In studies by Wood and Duffy (1966), Curlee (1969) and McLachlan *et al.* (1976), the middle-aged married housewife, not working outside her home, was found to be a higher consumer of alcohol in attempting to escape her isolation and loneliness.

Seligman's (1975) theory of learned helplessness exemplifies women's hopeless attitude which results in depression, withdrawal, and lack of motivation. There is growing awareness of the powerlessness of women in our male-dominated society, where women do not perceive that they have control over situations or that their actions bring rewards or recognition (LeDray and Chaignot, 1980; Guttentag *et al.*, 1980; Schaef, 1981). Belle's (1982) work with poor single mothers is a powerful documentation of their helplessness fighting an indifferent government system. Studies by Chodoff (1972) and Goldberg (1973) report of depressed women with 'helpless' characteristics, and are supported by Radloff and Monroe (1978), Notman *et al.* (1978) and Kivett (1979).

Miller (1976) states that women have been relegated to nurturing tasks and may be forced to decide between either personal growth or development of an intimate relationship with men. The problem of wife-battering has increasingly been brought to the attention of the American public. Claerhout *et al.* (1982) state that violence occurs in 35–50 per cent of all marital relationships and that in part cultural attitudes explain the occurrence. While men are taught to be aggressive and independent, women often assume dependent and submissive roles in marital relationships. Walker (1979) suggests that these victims of domestic violence typically have low self-esteem, chronic anxiety, learned helplessness, denial, shame, guilt and psychosomatic complaints. Many women are withdrawn, depressed, and use denial to alleviate high tension levels. Johnson (1979) states that these dependent women tend to be high suicide risks.

Depression is also theorized to result from an individual's own misinterpretation of losses and life events. That depressed women tend to see themselves and the world around them in a negative manner is consistent with Beck's (1978) cognitive theory. For example, their adjustment to aging in the American youth-oriented society, where aging is not accepted (Chenitz, 1979) and where negative stereotyping of aging abounds (Emery, 1981). Women's attitudes toward themselves reveal low self-esteem and fears of failure (Horney, 1967; Bardwick, 1978), passivity and dependency (Kagan and Moss, 1971; Cooperstock, 1979), and a tendency to be self-critical (Lowenthal and Chiriboga, 1972). All these symptoms are common to the syndrome of subclinical depression (Beck *et al.*, 1979).

Treatment and prevention

There are two concerns that remain with treatment and prevention issues. One is that traditional treatment approaches by male therapists perpetuate the passivity and negative self-image of women (Weissman and Klerman, 1977). The other is that while there are numerous programmes to treat depression, treatment usually begins after the depression has reached a serious level. This lack of early identification and intervention does not support nursing's commitment to prevention and health maintenance. Regarding the sex-role stereotyping, Broverman *et al.* (1970) concluded that professional therapists have described women clients as dependent, submissive, highly emotional, and less able to make important decisions than men. Brown and Hellinger (1975) found female therapists to have more understanding attitudes toward women patients. Kjervik and Palta (1978) identified the psychiatric nurse as the professional therapist who was least likely to hold stereotypic attitudes toward women.

Rationale for a nurse-facilitated group intervention

The apparent centrality of psychosocial factors to depression in women suggests that much might be done through early identification and treatment of symptoms through psychotherapeutic intervention. Once these women have been identified in urban and rural areas, growth-support groups can be established. At minimal expense these groups may provide the support necessary to develop and establish successful coping strategies for women while preventing more serious depression (Gordon and LeDray, 1985).

A group approach can be far superior to individual treatment for women in that it allows contact with peers who are likely to be dealing with some of the same role conflicts (Maykowsky, 1980). Coping strategies can be tested and shared within the supportive, safe environment of a group. These groups have been recognized as especially important in helping to lower the acknowledged sense of helplessness, powerlessness, and isolation of women living in communities (Davis, 1977). In 1981 van Servellen and Dull identified group therapy as an effective medium to promote positive change in self-esteem of depressed women. Dinnauer *et al.* (1981) emphasize the strength of groups as providing an important structure for women's social learning. Gallese and Treuting (1981) state that a women's group 'can be a lifesaver' for women feeling overwhelming stress, such as rape victims. The value of these groups goes far beyond their original purpose and provides the individuals with a sense of community (Back and Taylor, 1976).

Current literature has supported the professional nurse (minimum: baccalaureate prepared) as a facilitator of women's support groups. Loomis (1979) expected these nurses would function well as group leaders with their preparation in group dynamics and communication skills. Professional nurses (of whom 97.2 per cent in America are women) are the logical primary therapeutic change-agents in facilitating effective women's groups for the following reasons.

1. They are traditionally accepted by women as trusted, caring, and helpful health professionals.
2. Academically prepared, they understand both the physiological and psychological aspects of women.
3. They appreciate the women's significant influence and role within the family system.
4. They empathize with, rather than stereotype, the women's current problems within society.
5. They serve as a positive role model for women (Gordon, 1982).

Braillier (1980) stresses the need for holistic health practice in the expanding role of the professional nurse. She feels nurses are 'ideal' resources to practice the holistic health approach since they deal with mind–body–spiritual aspects with relative ease. Professional nurses are committed to health maintenance and prevention. The efficacy for involving the client as an active participant in this emerging holistic health movement across America has been stated by Tubesing *et al*. (1977).

Description of 1983 study of depressed women in Great Britain

. . .

Aim of study

The purpose of the study was to evaluate the effectiveness of a nurse-facilitated group intervention in the alleviation of depression in women of Great Britain.

The samples

Twenty women, 40–60 years of age, were selected for the study. These subjects had been recruited though a public service radio broadcast (BBC airwaves) seeking depressed women as participants. Preliminary screening took place during the eight-minute early morning public announcement by Gordon that in order for women to be eligible for the study they needed to be 40–60 years of age, they must speak English, and they should not presently be seeing a counsellor or psychiatrist. There was an overwhelming response to the broadcast from hundreds of women not only living in England but in areas as widespread as Wales, Belgium, Scotland, and France. The University of London's phone lines were flooded with calls, confirming the author's belief that depression in women is extensive. Over 200 women came to Chelsea College to meetings giving information about the study. Six meetings were scheduled at various hours of the week (i.e. Tuesdays 10 a.m., 3 p.m., and 7 p.m.; Fridays 10 a.m., 3 p.m. and 7 p.m.) to fit the plans of mothers and working women. Most women were working and came to the 7 p.m. meetings. Gordon (principal investigator) met the women in a large classroom where introductions were made and an overview of the study was given. Many women aged 20–30 years came to learn about the study and were disappointed that they were unable to participate until further group experiences were available. They shared feelings of depression. All interested women ($n = 119$) who met the criteria were assigned a code number, filled out a demographic questionnaire, signed a consent form, and were given two additional tests to further help the investigator screen these volunteers. The Beck Depression Inventory (Beck, 1978) and the SCL-90-R (Derogatis, 1976) were administered. Eighty-one women who scored 14–26 on the Beck test, indicating they were mildly to moderately depressed and who were also within 'normal limits' on the SCL-90-R (therefore were not psychotic, psychopathic or suicidal) were eligible to be group members. However, the study could only include 20 women, therefore the need for random selection was indicated. All (81) code numbers were placed in a box and the first ten numbers drawn out by a visiting psychologist were assigned to the control group, the second ten code numbers pulled out by this same psychologist were assigned to the experimental group. The following week all women who came to the information meeting were informed by letter of their inclusion or exclusion in the study. Eight women who showed no depression on the Beck's test were thanked but dismissed. Thirty women who showed severe depression on the Beck's test were given information about professional resource help. Of these thirty women, six were found to be most severely depressed and the investigator informed them by telephone that their initial tests indicated that they were very depressed. The women confirmed these test results and were cooperative about seeing their general practitioner the next day. All reported back to Gordon that they had been given medication and were under the direct supervision of their physicians.

Of the twenty selected subjects, all women were white, upper middle class, with a mean age of 51 years. Eight women were married and had children, while one was divorced, five were separated, four were single, and two were widowed. Twelve women were working, one was unemployed, while seven were homemakers. Demographic differences in the experimental and control groups appeared incidental regarding age, marital status, working full-time or part-time.

Instruments used in the study

For selection of subjects

Beck depression inventory This inventory (Beck, 1978) is a 21-item, self-report measure (range = 0–63) used to measure level of depression. The internal consistency and validity of this widely used instrument has been well documented (Beck and Beamesderfer, 1974; Shaw, 1977). The score of 14–22 is in the mild–moderate depressed range and was chosen to obtain a sample of subjects.

Test–retest stability (97 cases) over a 1 week interval was high (r = 0.86 to 0.93) and the measure appears sensitive to spontaneous or treatment related change (Beck, 1972). There was a correlation coefficient of 0.75 between the Beck test and Hamilton Rating Scale (Schwab *et al.*, 1967). The instrument was highly effective in discriminating between depression and anxiety (Beck, 1978).

The SCL-90-R inventory This inventory (Derogatis, 1976) is a 90-item self-report measure (norm T score = 50, SC = 10) used to screen for pathology and suicide risk. Designed to reflect nine psychological symptoms (obsessive–compulsive, somatization, paranoid ideation, psychoticism, depression, anxiety, hostility, phobic anxiety and interpersonal sensitivity) seen in psychiatric patients. Measures of internal consistency were obtained from 219 hospitalized volunteers. Alpha coefficients ranged from 0.77 to 0.90 for the dimension scores. Test–retest coefficient for 94 psychiatric outpatients (over a 1 week interval) ranged from 0.80 to 0.90. The SCL-90-R correlated high 0.88 with the Minnesota Multiphasic Personality Inventory. With the Middlesex Hospital Questionnaire, six symptom dimensions were contrasted, aggregate score correlation was 0.92 (Derogatis, 1976). The SCL-90-R was chosen as the one-time assessment measure for these depressed women because of the need to eliminate from the study those who did show symptoms of psychosis, psychopathology and suicide risk.

Pre- and post-test (Comparison of control–experimental groups)

Coopersmith's self-esteem inventory This inventory (Ryden, 1978) is a 58-item self-report used to measure self-esteem in adult subjects. Test was found to have a test–retest reliability of 0.80 for 32 women over periods of 6–58 weeks. The high level of stability over a period of 58 weeks reinforces the idea that the evolutive aspect of one's concept of self, as reflected in self-report, has a considerable degree of consistency over time. Because self-esteem may be related to a person's depression, Ryden's modification of the Coopersmith's self-esteem inventory was chosen to measure the subject's self-esteem.

The social adjustment self-report The SAS (Weissman and Paykel, 1974) is a 42-item instrument that measures overall social adjustment as well as performance in six major areas of functioning: work, family, social roles, etc. Self-report results based on 76 depressed out-patients were comparable to those obtained from relatives as well as by a rater who interviewed the patient directly. This measure was validated using depressed out-patients and is capable of discriminating between recovered patients and those in acute stages of illness. Validity data show that the instrument correlates highly with independent ratings of overall social adjustment made by mental health professionals ($r = 0.72$) and by significant others ($r = 0.74$). The SAS is also sensitive to change and yields significant differences in scores before and after treatment (Bothwell and Weissman, 1977).

Life experience survey The purpose of the LES (Sarason *et al.*, 1978) is to measure life changes. Advantages of this 57-item measure are that it allows for separation of positive and negative life experiences as well as individualized ratings of the impact of events. Test–retest reliability (at 5–6 weeks) is 0.56–0.88. Correlations with social desirability were -0.05 to 0.01 showing good discriminative validity. Correlations with illness, although low (0.3–0.4), are consistent with other stress measures. The LES was chosen for this study to help identify and measure stress areas of women subjects.

The young loneliness inventory The YLS (Young, 1981) is a 19-item self-report inventory used to diagnose the severity of recent loneliness. Various test items assess the client's relationship with friends and close family members during a given period of time, by rating on a scale of 0 (low) to 3 (high) the *frequency, disclosure, caring* and *physical intimacy* they experienced in each relationship. Young establishes cutting scores as 8–9 (normal), 10–18 (mild), 19–29 moderate to severe, 30 high, and 50 as a very high degree of loneliness. The YLS has been tested for reliability and validity with both out-patient, college, and university populations. In assessing reliability, measures of consistency were obtained with these populations. Alpha coefficients ranged from 0.78 in the college to 80 in the university, to 0.84 in the mood clinic, and were considered reasonably high.

Beck depression inventory – 'significant other' form The BDI has been adapted for completion by significant other(s) of the identified patient (Hollon, 1980). All 21 items from the original inventory have been left intact other than being worded in third person, and scoring principles are identical to those for the self-report form. While little validity data are yet available for the 'significant other' form of the BDI, initial information indicated that test provides a reasonably satisfactory means of assessing depression.

Pre-post-testing

All subjects (n = 20) were given the five self-report tests described (Cooper-smith's Self-Esteem, Weissman's Social Adjustment Scale, Young's Loneliness Scale, Sarason's Life Experience Survey and the Beck Depression test filled out by a 'significant other') before the first group session started and after the four-teenth group session was over. Test scores from the control group and experi-mental groups were compared and changes in levels of depression, self-esteem and loneliness, etc. were analysed.

Procedure

Group sessions

After meeting screening criteria (over radio and at the information meet-ing) subjects were randomly assigned to either the experimental (treatment, n = 10) or control (no-treatment, n = 10) condition. The treatment consisted of 14 weekly (2-hour) group sessions led by two professional nurses with group experience (one psychiatric nurse expert came highly recommended from Maudsley Hospital, London, one nurse with a Master's degree in psy-chiatric nursing came from USA). These nurses were briefly orientated on the structured group intervention, which utilized a holistic health approach with concepts from the cognitive–behaviour–affective models. The nurse facili-tators were provided with a training manual the contents of which included group dynamics, reinforcement theory, and evaluation of group process. Lecture content with specific objectives and discussion questions for each of the fourteen group sessions was also included in the training manual.

The experimental group

Women in the experimental group chose to meet at 7–9 p.m. on Monday evenings in a comfortable room at Chelsea College (May–August 1983). The setting was located in a convenient, safe area of London. Some women came by car but most of them came by bus or subway trains.

During the first two sessions each woman was given equal time to 'tell her story'. After that second session repeated recounting of problems was not encouraged. The structure of group sessions devoted the first hour to lecture, education, and discussion, while the second hour was spent in activities related to the session topic. Each woman was provided with a workbook and was expected to come to the group sessions with assigned homework com-pleted. Weekly topics included content found in the women's workbook: goal setting, signs and symptoms of depression, cognitions and feelings, self-worth, building relationships, communication skills, assertiveness, conflict management and decision making, stress, relaxation, exercise, nutrition, menstruation/menopause and strength building.

All group sessions were tape-recorded for the first three sessions but this was discontinued due to inability to hear voices clearly. The women were delighted to see the tape-recorder removed.

The control group

Women assigned to the control condition received no intervention between pre- and post-testing. At the first information meeting they had been asked to refrain from joining other therapy groups or seeking counselling while the study was going on unless necessary. Eight women in the control condition expressed a desire to be included in later group sessions if others were to be offered.

Results

Analysis of the data

There were no significant mean pre-treatment differences between the two treatment conditions on any of the five self-report tests, indicating that the randomization procedure was successful.

Because estimation of 'raw change' scores as measures of effectiveness of a treatment is subject to difficulties in interpretation (Cronbach and Furby, 1970), the Cohen and Cohen (1975) procedure for analysis of partial variance was used to assess the effectiveness of the treatment programme.

Statistically significant post-test differences between the control and treatment groups were demonstrated for depression, self-esteem and hopelessness. Over 35 per cent of the variance in post-test depression scores was linearly accounted for by the pre-test depression scores. Once the effects of pre-test were removed, the treatment condition accounted for approximately 40.4 per cent of the variance in regressed change in depression from pre-test to post-test ($F = (1,17) = 11.52$, $p < 0.025$). Adjustments for unreliability of the depression measure using a reliability estimate of 0.86 also resulted in significant differences between the control and treatment groups ($F = (1,17) = 13.41$, $p < 0.005$). This difference represented almost one full standard deviation difference in post-test depression scores for the two groups and a classification difference from 'mild-moderate' to 'mild' on Beck's inventory.

Statistically significant improvement in scores on Coopersmith's Self-Esteem Inventory was also demonstrated for subjects in the treatment condition in comparison to those in the control group. While 54 per cent of the variance in post-test self-esteem scores could be linearly accounted for by pre-test levels of self-esteem, approximately 58.8 per cent of the variance in regressed change from pre-test to post-test was accounted for by treatment condition ($F = (1,17) = 24.23$, $p < 0.001$). Adjustments for unreliability of the self-esteem measure using 0.80 as an estimate of reliability yielded even higher statistically significant results ($F = (1,17) = 56.92$, $p < 0.001$). Mean post-test scores adjusted for unreliability and pre-test performance were 63.78 for the treatment group and 48.12 for the control group. Again, the treatment group was almost one full standard deviation above the control group in post-test self-esteem level.

Feelings of hopelessness were also significantly reduced between pre-test and post-test for the treatment subjects, whereas there was an increase in these feelings for the control group over the same period. Over 20 per cent of the variance in post-test hopelessness scores was accounted for by pre-test feelings of hopelessness and 45.2 per cent of the variance in regressed change in hopelessness scores was accounted for by the treatment manipulation $(F = (1,17) = 14.01, p < 0.005)$. No direct reliability estimates for the Beck Hopelessness Scale were available so a reliability of 0.80 was assumed. Adjustments to the analysis based upon this level of reliability resulted in higher levels of statistical significance $(F = (1,17) = 20.81, p < 0.001)$. Subjects in the treatment group $(X = 5.76)$ scored over six units below the subjects in the control group $(X = 11.82)$. This difference between treatment and control groups represented over one standard deviation difference in performance.

Similar analyses were applied to the remaining dependent measures. No statistically significant differences between control and treatment groups on the post-test measures for loneliness, depression as rated by a significant other, social adjustment or anxiety level were observed. Perhaps the 14-week time interval for the study was not a sufficient time period to observe significant changes on these variables. Also, the significant other form of the Beck Depression Inventory is not as valid as the self-report form and, generally, measures of depression by significant others tend to underestimate self-report measures of depression. Both of these could have affected the results of the study.

The findings suggest that nurse-facilitated groups do provide a therapeutic value to moderately depressed women. The 14-week time interval was sufficient to demonstrate improvement in subjects' feelings of self-esteem and reduction in their feelings of depression and hopelessness. It seems reasonable that improvement in a woman's feelings of self-esteem and self-concept could potentially stress other aspects of her life as she learned to cope with her new sense of being and with others in her life. Also, it is possible that others, especially significant others in her life, must also learn to adapt to a woman with higher feelings of self-esteem. Perhaps this accounts for the lack of significant change in the feelings of loneliness, social adjustment, and anxiety observed in this study. Further studies should investigate this possibility.

Condensed data in notebooks

Observation notes were carefully written by both nurse group-facilitators after each session. The date, the number of members present, and the reactions of members relating to lateness or absence of peers were recorded in notebooks. Individual verbal/non-verbal behaviour was described, as well as indications of group stages, themes, and cohesiveness observed. The group met during summer 1983.

The wealth of information emerging from the content of the notebooks was too great to be included in this single chapter, however specific data observed during each session is described. Names have been changed for confidentiality.

Session 1

All women arrived on time, except Diane who had 'forgotten' about a previous engagement. All members were well dressed, neat. They looked like serious business women as introductions were made. Everyone was polite and interested. During the nurse's explanation of expectations for group leaders and members, rules of confidentiality, etc. most women sat with folded arms and guarded facial expressions. After tea and coffee, the members seemed to feel more relaxed with the two nurses gently inviting more trust. Many questions indicating anxiety about their own expectations of the group sessions arose. There was denial of feelings, i.e. 'Well, there really isn't much to talk about,' or 'Oh, I couldn't talk about anger because I have never felt it.' Two women felt there was danger in becoming 'too introspective'. Several shared their loathing of lies. Themes: mistrust, anger, sadness, and some wonder of 'how "things" at home can really change'.

Session 2

All women were punctual. With little hesitation they went into talking about their life problems. There were 'moving' moments as the women revealed their suffering and how they had suppressed a lot of their own feelings for the 'good of the family'. Support for each other was evident, i.e. 'Yes, I know what you mean, I felt that pain too when my children left home.' Women appeared more positive, they said they looked forward to coming to the group, i.e. 'Its good that there are others we can talk to.' Themes: marriage vs career, the freedom and the frustrations of living alone. Stages: trust, some cohesiveness, i.e. use of 'we' instead of 'me'.

Session 3

Nearly everyone was talking at once. Much discussion, 'advice giving'. The group felt very charged and intense, with great sharing of deep losses, personal failures in life. Several spoke of painful separation from family when sent to boarding schools. Facilitators felt exhausted after the session and were concerned that 'too much was shared too early'.

Session 4

The group was dominated by Lisa who spent a great deal of time on frivolous events in her life; there was much chit-chat and unheeded advice giving. Nurse-facilitators found themselves irritated that the group was not 'moving', that there seemed to be a conscious avoidance of sharing deep feelings ...

perhaps too painful from the last session. Nurses did intervene, taking control of the storytelling and the women grew thoughtful. Themes: loneliness, feelings of low self-worth, loss of male companionship.

Session 5

Three members were absent. The group appeared quiet, serious, more of a 'working' group. More intimacy emerged, e.g. how they felt powerless in marital relationships with their husbands who 'did what they wanted'. Tremendous denial of their anger toward others. They tended to blame themselves that their children did not meet their expectations, that they were concerned and hurt how their children reacted to relatives, friends. Stage: intimacy.

Session 6

Again much 'advice giving' (how to lose weight, etc.) was apparent, and facilitators needed to get the group back to talking about the assigned homework on discussing feelings. It was a very productive session with much clarification of negative and positive feelings, of how 'should', 'ought', 'must' thinking causes their feelings of hopelessness. One woman shared how hard it was being the 'other' woman in a relationship and received support and understanding.

Session 7

Homework assignment related to learning how difficult it was to learn how to be assertive. They said they were 'brought up' to be nice, lovely ladies and it was easier to remain passive. They found it most difficult to be aggressive and nearly impossible to be assertive. Some 'pairing off' by group members, some non-direct hostility toward a domineering member.

Session 8

'Entire group came looking very pretty tonight', wrote one nurse-facilitator. The women initiated discussion on the value of the group. One woman had been turned down twice that week for jobs, but had looked forward to coming to the group for support. Much sincere feedback and support was evident. Karen said she could take what she learned in each group session and apply it daily. Facilitators felt sad and shared these feelings with the group: many women had said that this group was the 'only' place they felt they could speak freely and easily. Stage: cohesiveness, group running itself.

Session 9

Vera was leaving the group for a new job in Southeast Asia. Fears and anxieties were expressed by Vera. All members told her they were happy for her, sad for themselves, and a bit envious of her new adventure. She thanked them for their caring and was taking her Women's Workbook with her. Again when advice was given to various members Elaine expressed frustration that members weren't allowing self-decision-making. Reactions were highly defended and difficult. Facilitators felt the group seemed blocked and permitted power struggles.

Session 10

No absences. Group members seemed much more serious, using workbooks, reflecting more on their own reactions to daily stress. Both nurses wrote: 'These women are bright, of high intelligence, and gain insight with relative ease.' Lisa appears to have learned constructive ways of dealing with conflicts regarding her employer. More women said they had more energy and more interest in life.

Session 11

Much discussion on feelings of failure as mothers. Expressions of anger, guilt. There was beginning talk about how sad it was that the group would soon come to an end. Reflections about Vera separating from them to go to Asia brought out an atmosphere of sombre mellowness. Peggy shared for the first time that she was chemically dependent. The group was surprised at this, but supported her for continuing to come to group and work on her low self-esteem. Women went on to discuss the problem of being divorced and having no job skills. (This is a similiar problem of middle-aged women in the United States.)

Session 12

Much talk of guilt when they say 'no' to doing favours for others and what to do about that guilt. Some pressure on facilitators to come up with answers. Many spoke of resistance to physical exercise. Some insight on how they resist change throughout their lives and it brings them depression. 'It is hard to change our habits.' Good discussion on the fears of taking risks to change. Definite cohesiveness between members . . . women see the facilitators as members.

Session 13

Discussion of menstruation and menopause evoked feelings of the loss of childbearing ability for some members. Support was given to each other. Others spoke of the pains of motherhood. One shared how much the group had helped her to see her children more objectively, to give them freedom to be adults, and be more accepting of her son and his 'unconventional' behaviour. She said she felt much happier in herself and that she couldn't have achieved that without help of the group. Afterwards group facilitators felt frustrated because there had not been enough time to discuss the sexual conflicts alluded to by several members.

Session 14

The last group centred on sexuality: both strategies for building positive and intimate sexual relationships, as well as sources for sexual conflict were discussed. Some women described sexual conflicts with their lovers or husbands, others explained their relationships lacked all sexual intimacy. It was interesting to observe how relaxed most of the women were discussing such personal problems. The last half hour of this session was used for group evaluation and feedback. The women felt sad that it was their last group because they felt that they had learned to trust and confide in each other. One member said she had never considered that the group would end. There was a consensus of opinion by all members and facilitators that the number of group meetings should be expanded to at least 20 sessions, so that the women would have more time to learn and test the coping skills they needed in meeting their daily problems. Facilitators felt more time was needed for termination. All the women described the groups as helpful, insightful, and supportive. They hoped to remain in touch with each other and there was an exchange of addresses. The women also gave cards and gifts to the nurses, who felt it was a wonderful experience for them. All left with much handshaking, some hugging, and tear-filled eyes.

Summary and implications for nursing

The widespread incidence of depression in women is identified as a major health problem in the world today. Prominent researchers report that women are twice as likely as men to suffer from depression. This chapter provides documentation of the stress factors that occur in women's daily lives which stem from social, family, and cultural demands on them. Women are still regarded as 'second-class' citizens with society's expectation that they are caretakers of men and children first while their own potential for self-actualization is disregarded. A consequence of this lack of recognition decreases women's self-fulfilment and self-worth. Women are the most underutilized talent in the world. Their sensitivity, creativeness, management skills, and enduring strength in crisis is taken for granted and undervalued. As a result they have feelings of frustration, inadequacy, and low self-esteem. Close relationships with significant others are of utmost importance to women. It is around attachment issues, more than any other sorts of issues, that depressive episodes in women tend to emerge. Women invest highly in intimate relationships with men and their children and to fail in those relationships, or to have them end becomes equated with failing in everything. Conflicts with husbands, children, in-laws, and lovers are cited by women as principal causes for their depression.

Depressed women in America have increased medical costs due to their repeated visits to physicians for psychosomatic complaints, chemical dependency, unnecessary gynaecological surgery, and high admissions to psychiatric hospital units. Due to the rising cost of health care, treatment approaches need to be efficacious, safe and cost-effective. . . .

Preliminary studies were conducted in the United States with thirty-eight women (40–60 years of age) as subjects. The purpose of the studies was to evaluate the effectiveness of a group intervention facilitated by professional nurses in alleviating depression in women. Pre-post-testing revealed that women who attended the structured group sessions showed a significant reduction in depression and a significant increase in self-esteem. In addition the participants' support and commitment to the group was demonstrated by high attendance to group sessions and their continued networking after the group sessions were over. Findings support the view that mild depression may lift over a period of 6–8 weeks and that replication of the study should include moderately depressed women.

The third study, a replication of the intervention model, was conducted in the University of London with twenty moderately depressed middle-aged women. These volunteers were randomly selected and assigned to either the experimental or control condition. The treatment consisted of 14 weekly (2-hour) structured group sessions led by two professional nurses in London. Detailed description of methodology, findings as well as nurses' observation by the group's nurse-facilitators are included in the chapter. Again, statistically significant post-test differences between control and experimental groups were demonstrated for depression, self-esteem and hopelessness.

The following conclusions emerge:

1. Professional nurses (baccalaureate graduates) tend to be effective facilitators of depressed women's groups. Nurses' abilities to help women has been substantiated in these studies in the USA and the UK.
2. That coping strategies for women can be taught, tested and shared within a supportive group atmosphere.
3. That replication of the intervention model with increased numbers of women of a variety of ages and background could be useful future nursing research.

The significance of the intervention model is:

1. To help women cope effectively, take an active role in their own health.
2. To prevent possible severe depression in women.
3. To gain data about the complex phenomena of depression in women.
4. To strengthen the family unit by increased self-esteem of women.

Use of this approach by nurses already available in the community to provide women this assistance (by use of provided instruction manuals for the group facilitators as well as for each woman) could also reduce health care costs.

References

Back, K. W. and Taylor, R. (1976). Self-help groups: tool or symbol? *Journal of Applied Behavioural Science*, **12**, 295–309.

Bardwick, J. M. (1978). Middle age and a sense of future. *Merrill-Palmer Quarterly*, **24**, 130–136.

Barrett, N. (1979). 'Women in the job market: occupations, earnings and career opportunities', in (ed. R. Smith). *The Subtle Revolution: Women at Work* Urban Institute, Washington, D.C.

Bart, P. B. (1971). 'Depression in middle-aged Women', in *Women in Sexist Society* (eds V. Gomich and B. Moran), pp. 163–186. Basic Books, New York.

Beck, A. T. (1972). 'Measuring depression: the depression inventory; *Recent Advances in the Psychobiology of the Depressive Illnesses* (In T. A. Williams, M. N. Katz and J. A. Shield). Government Printing Office, Washington, D.C.

Beck, A. .T. (1978). *Depression: Causes and Treatment*, pp. 12–43, 186–207. University of Pennsylvania Press, Philadelphia, PA.

Beck, A. T. and Beamesderfer, A. (1974). 'Assessment of depression, the depression inventories', in *Psychological Measurements in Psychopharmacology and Modern Pharmacopsychiatry* (ed. P. Pichot), Vol. 7. Karger, Basle.

Beck, A. T., Rush, A. J., Shaw, B. F. and Emery G. (1979). *Cognitive Therapy of Depression*. Guilford Press, New York.

Belle, D. (1982). *Lives in Stress: Women and Depression*. Sage Publications, Beverly Hills, CA.

Bothwell, S. and Weissman, M. (1977). Social impairments four years after an acute depressive episode. *American Journal of Orthopsychiatry*, **47**, 231–237.

Brailler, L. (1980). 'Holistic health practice: expanding the role of the psychiatric-mental health nurse', in *Community Mental Health Nursing* (ed. J. Lancaster). Mosby, New York.

Broverman, I. K., Broverman, D., Clarkson, F. E., Rosendrantz, P. and Vogel, S. R. (1970). Sex-role stereotypes and clinical judgments of mental health. *Journal of Counselling and Clinical Psychology*, **34**, 1–7.

Brown, C. R. and Hellinger, M. L. (1975). Therapists' attitudes toward women. *Social Work*, **21**, 266–270.

Brown, G. W., Bhrolchain M. N. and Harris, T. (1975). Social class and psychiatric disturbance among women in an urban population. *Sociology*, **9**, 225–254.

Carmen, E., Russo, N. F. and Miller, J. B. (1981). Inequality and women's mental health: an overview. *American Journal of Psychiatry*, **138**, 1319–1330.

Chenitz, W. C. (1979). Primary depression in older women: are current theories and treatment of depression relevant to this age group? *Journal of Psychiatric Nursing and Mental Health Services*, 17–23.

Cherlin, A. J. (1981). *Marriage, Divorce, Remarriage*. Harvard University Press, Boston, MA.

Chodoff, P. (1972). The depressive personality. *Archives of General Psychiatry*, **27**, 666–673.

Claerhout, S., Elder, J. and Carolyn, J. (1982). Problem-solving skills of rural battered women. *American Journal of Community Psychology*, **10**(5), 605–606.

Clayton, P. J., Martin, S., Davis, M. and Wochnik, E. (1980). Mood disorders in women professionals. *Journal of Affective Disorders*, **2**, 37–46.

Cohen, J. and Cohen, P. (1975). *Applied Multiple Regression/Correlation Analysis for the Behavioral Sciences*, pp. 378–393. Wiley, New York.

Cooperstock, R. (1979). A review of women's psychotropic drug use. *Canadian Journal of Psychiatry*, **24**, 29–34.

Cronbach, L. J. and Furby, L. (1970). How should we measure 'change' – or should we? *Psychological Bulletin*, **74**, 68–80.

Curlee, (1969). Alcoholism and the 'empty nest'. *Bulletin of Menninger Clinic*, **33**, 165–170.

Davis, S. M. (1977). Women's liberation groups as a primary preventive mental health strategy. *Community Mental Health Journal*, **13**, 219–228.

Derogatis, L. (1976). *SCL-90 (Revised Version) Manual-1*. Johns Hopkins University School of Medicine, Baltimore, MD. 21205.

Dinnauer, L., Miller, M. and Frankforter, M. (1981). Implementation strategies for an inpatient woman's support group. *Journal of Psychiatric Nursing and Mental Health Services*, **19**, 13–16.

Dohrenwend, B. S. (1973). Social status and stressful life events. *Journal of Personality and Social Psychology*, **28**, 225–235.

Editorial (1979). Hysterectomy and the quality of a woman's life. *Archives of International Medicine*, **139**, 146.

Emery, G. (1981). *A New Beginning: How You Can Change Your Life Through Cognitive Therapy*. Simon and Schuster, New York.

Fiske, D. W., Hunt, H. F., Luborsky, L., Orne, T. M., Parloff, M. B., Reiser, M. F. and Tuma, A. H. (1970). Planning of research on effectiveness of psychotherapy. *Archives of General Psychiatry*, **22**, 22.

Gallese, L. and Treuting, E. (1981). Help for rape victims through group therapy. *Journal of Psychiatric Nursing and Mental Health Services*, **19**, 20–21.

Goldberg, A. (1973). Psychotherapy of narcissistic injuries. *Archives of General Psychiatry*, **28**, 722–726.

Gordon, V. C. (1979). 'Women and divorce: implications for nursing care,' in *Women in Stress: A Nursing Perspective*, (ed. O. O. Kjervik-Martinson), pp. 259–276. Appleton-Century-Croft, New York.

Gordon, V. C. (1982). Themes and cohesives observed in a depressed women's support group. *Issues in Mental Health Nursing*, **4**, 115–125.

Gordon, V. and LeDray, L. (1985). Depression in women: the challenge of treatment and prevention. *Journal of Psychosocial Nursing and Mental Health Services*, **23**, 26–34.

Gove, W. (1972). The relationship between sex roles, mental illness and marital status. *Social Forces*, **51**, 34–44.

Guttentag, M., Slasin, S. and Belle, D. (1980). *The Mental Health of Women*, pp. 21–30, 57–89. Academic Press, New York.

Hirschfield, R. M. (1980). In *Unfinished Business: Pressure Points in the Lives of Women* (ed. M. Scarf), p. 277. Ballatine Books, New York.

Hollon, S. O. (1980). Beck's 'Significant Other' Form (unpublished).

Horney, K. (1967). *Feminine Psychology*, pp. 124–132. W. W. Norton, New York.

Johnson, K. K. (1979). Durkheim revisited: why do women kill themselves? *Suicide and Life Threatening Behaviour*, **9**, 145–153.

Kagan, J. and Moss, H. A. (1971). 'Birth to maturity', in *Psychology of Women* (ed. J. M. Bardwick). Harper & Row, New York.

Kaslow, S. (1982). Marriage and intimacy: The surprising staying power of loveless marriages. *Ladies Home Journal*, **3**, 41–48.

Kivett, V. R. (1979). Religious motivation in middle age: correlates and implications. *Journal of Gerontology*, **34**, 106–115.

Kjervik, D. K. and Palta, M. (1978). Sex-role stereotyping in assessments of mental health. *Nursing Research*, **27**, 166–171.

LeDray, L. and Chaignot, M. (1980). Services of sexual assault victims in Hennepin County. *Evaluation and Change* (special issue) 131–134.

Lewinsohn, P., Sullivan, J. and Grosscup, S. (1982). 'Behavioral therapy: clinical applications', in *Short Term Psychotherapies of Depression* (ed. A. J. Rush), pp. 50–87. The Guilford Press, New York.

Loomis, M. E. (1979). *Group Process for Nurses*, Vol. 23, pp. 146–147. Mosby, St. Louis, MD.

Lopata, H. Z. (1971). Widows as a minority group. *The Gerontologist*, Spring, 67–75.

Lowenthal, M. F. and Chiriboga, D. (1972). Transition to the empty nest: crisis, challenge or relief? *Archives of General Psychiatry*, 26, 8–14.

Martin, R. L., Roberts, W. V. and Clayton, P. J. (1980). Psychiatric status after hysterectomy. *Journal of the American Medical Association*, 244, 350–353:

Maykowsky, V. P. (1980). 'Stress and mental health of women: a discussion of research and issues', in *The Mental Health of Women* (ed. M. Guttentag). Academic Press, New York.

McLachlan, J. F., R. L. Walderman, D. F. Birchmore and Marsden, L. R. (1976). Self-evaluation, role satisfaction in the woman alcoholic. *The International Journal of Addictions*, 14(6), 809–832.

Miller, J. (1976). *Toward A New Psychology of Women*, pp. 64–73. Beacon Press, Boston, MA.

Neuberry, P., Weissman, M. and Myers, J. (1979). Working wives and housewives: do they differ in mental status and social adjustment? *American Journal of Orthopsychiatry*, 49, 282–290.

Neugarten, B., Wood, L., Krainer, R. and Loomis, B. (1963). Women's attitudes toward the menopause. *Vita Humana*, 6, 140–151.

Notman, M. (1979). Midlife concerns in women: implications of the menopause. *American Journal of Psychiatry*, 136, 1270–1274.

Notman, M., Nadelson, C. and Bennett, M. (1978). Achievement conflict in women. *Psychotherapy and Psychosomatics*, 29, 203–213.

Parloff, M. B. (1980). Psychotherapy and research: an anaclitic depression. *Psychiatry*, 43, 280.

Pilisuk, M. and Froland, C. (1978). Kinship, social network, social support and health. *Social Science and Medicine*, 12(B), 273–280.

Powell, B. (1977). The empty nest, employment, and psychiatric symptoms in college-educated women. *Psychology of Women Quarterly*, 2, 35–43.

Radloff, L. (1975). Sex differences in depression: the effects of occupation and marital status. *Sex Roles*, 1, 249–264.

Radloff, L. and Monroe, M. (1978). 'Sex differences in helplessness – with implications for depression', in *Career Development and Counseling of Women* (ed. L. Hansen and R. Rapoza), pp. 199–204. Thomas, Springfield, II.

Radloff, L. S. and Rae, D. (1979). Susceptibility and precipitating factors in depression: sex differences and similarities. *Journal of Abnormal Psychology*, 88, 174–181.

Raphael, B. (1976). 'Psychiatric aspects of hysterectomy', in *Modern Perspectives in the Psychiatric Aspects of Surgery* (ed. J. G. Howell), p. 425. Brunner-Mazel, New York.

Ryden, M. (1978). Coopersmith self-esteem inventory (adult version). *Psychological Reports*, 43, 1189–1980.

Sarason, I., Johnson, J. and Siegel, J. (1978). Assessing the impact of life changes: development of the Life Experiences Survey. *Journal of Consulting and Clinical Psychology*, 46, 932–946.

Scarf, M. (1980). *Unfinished Business: Pressure Points in the Lives of Women*, pp. 442–448. Ballantine Books, New York.

Schaef, A. W. (1981). *Women's Reality*. Winston Press, Minneapolis, MN.

Schwab, J. J., Bralow, M. and Holzer, C. (1967). A comparison of two rating scales for depression. *Journal of Clinical Psychology*, **23**, 94–96.

Seligman, M. E. (1975). *Helplessness*. W. H. Freeman, San Francisco, CA.

Shaw, B. F. (1977). Comparison of cognitive therapy and behavior therapy in the treatment of depression. *Journal of Consulting and Clinical Psychology*, **45**, 543–551.

Shields, L. (1980). *Displaced Homemakers*. McGraw-Hill, New York.

Stevenson, J. (1977). *Issues and Crises During Middlescence*, pp. 165, 168–186, 216. Appleton-Century-Crofts, New York.

Thurnher, M. (1976). Midlife marriage: sex differences in evaluation and perspectives. *International Journal of Aging and Human Development*, **7**, 129–135.

Tubesing, D., Holinger, P., Westberg, G. and Lichter, E. (1977). The Wholistic Health Center Project. *Medical Care*, **15**, 217–227.

Tucker, S. J. (1977). The menopause: How much soma and how much psyche? *JOGN Nursing*, **6**, 40–47.

van Keep, P. and Prill, H. (1975). Psycho-sociology of menopause and post-menopause. *Frontiers in Hormone Research*, **3**, 32–39.

van Servellen, G. and Dull, L. (1981). Group psychotherapy for depressed women: a model. *Journal of Psychiatric Nursing and Mental Health Services*, **19**, 25–30.

Walker, L. E. (1979). *The Battered Woman*. Harper & Row, New York.

Weissman, M. M. and Paykel, E. S. (1974). *The Depressed Woman*. University of Chicago Press, Chicago, IL.

Weissman, M. M. and Klerman, G. L. (1977). Sex differences and the epidemiology of depression. *Archives of General Psychiatry*, **34**, 98–111.

Weissman, M., Pincus, C., Radding, N., Lawrence, R. and Siegel, R. (1973). The educated housewife: mild depression and the search for work. *American Journal Orthopsychiatry*, **43**(4), 565–573.

Wittenborn, J. R. and Buhler, R. (1979). Somatic discomforts among depressed women. *Archives of General Psychiatry*, **36**, 465–471.

Wood, H. P. and Duffy, E. L. (1966). Psychological factors in alcoholic women. *American Journal of Psychiatry*, **123**(3), 341–345.

Young, J. E. (1981). 'Cognitive therapy and loneliness', in (eds *New Directions in Cognitive Therapy*, pp. 139–159. G. Emery, S. Hollon, and R. Bedrosian). Guilford Press, New York.

## 9

Health visitors' and social workers' perceptions of child-care problems

Robert Dingwall and Susan Fox

Need health visitors be nurses? This is one of those questions which keeps cropping up in the professional press without ever achieving a definite resolution. In part, of course, this question is too vague for any firm answer to be given. It all depends upon what we want health visitors to do and how we propose to train them. A more sensible question, however, might be to ask what difference a nursing background makes to health visitors. Does it actually have such a distinctive effect on their practice that we should insist on its being maintained? In attempting to answer this we do, of course, face the obvious methodological difficulty of being unable to compare nursing- and non-nursing-trained health visitors doing exactly the same work. Nevertheless, there are significant areas of overlap between the work of health visitors and of other health and welfare occupations. By comparing their approaches to these areas we may get some indication of the extent to which a nursing background does influence health visiting practice.

This chapter describes a preliminary attempt to explore this question by adapting techniques developed by Giovannoni and Becerra (1979) to study variations in professional and lay definitions of child mistreatment in the United States. Their approach is used to examine the degree to which there are differences in the perception of child-care problems between health visitors and social workers in one English town. If such differences can be indentified, we can then consider whether they could be explained in terms of the different background and training of the two occupations. It is not claimed that this study is representative of national experience, but we do hope to establish the value of the approach and to show that the results are sufficiently interesting to justify further investigation.

Defining child mistreatment

Giovannoni and Becerra's original study was designed to examine the extent of agreement between members of different occupations in health and welfare work about what should be defined as child abuse or neglect, and how seriously particular instances should be regarded. The study was based on a sample drawn from four occupational groups in the Los Angeles area – 71 lawyers, 79 paediatricians, 50 police officers and 113 social workers. (In a subsequent phase these groups were also compared with a sample of the general population.) Each respondent was asked to rate a set of one or two sentence vignettes describing incidents which might be definable as mistreatment of a child. These vignettes were derived from the professional literature, recorded cases in law and local practice and the authors' own experience. They can be broadly classified into those concerned with parental role failure in the physical care of the child (e.g. nutritional neglect, medical neglect, poor supervision, inattention to cleanliness, clothing and housing) and those concerned with other caretaker responsibilities (e.g. fostering delinquency, emotional mistreatment, alcohol and drugs, parental sexual mores and educational neglect). Within each category the vignettes depicted incidents varying in severity. In all, 78 pairs of vignettes were used, one of each pair being a simple description of an incident, the other adding a statement of the consequences. Information was also collected relating to the respondents' age, sex and experience of child-rearing, to investigate whether such personal characteristics influenced definitions of mistreatment in a way which transcended occupational training or experience. The authors found significant differences in the responses to 69 of the 78 vignettes, although there were also considerable areas of agreement between members of particular occupations.

The vignette technique

For this study 20 vignettes were selected from the 156 (78 pairs) used by Giovannoni and Becerra. The selection was designed to include examples from each of the response clusters identified through a factor analysis. (Details of this procedure can be found in their monograph, pp. 144–156.) From each cluster we included the items which yielded the largest variation in responses between U.S. social workers and U.S. paediatricians. Although there are, of course, great differences between health visitors and paediatricians, it was felt that this selection would maximize the chances of polarizing the respondents in our study between 'medical' and 'social' definitions of mistreatment, if such polarities were to be found. The vignettes (V1–V20) are set out in Table 9.1. Their phrasing was unchanged from the originals except to replace the American words 'yard' and 'garbage' by the English 'garden' and 'refuse', in V18 and V20, respectively.

In the original study, respondents were asked to rate each vignette according to its implications for a 7-year-old child. The present study modified this to a 4-year-old. This reflects the health visitors' particular responsibilities for children under 5 and, in our view, made it possible for both groups to draw equally directly on their own professional experience.

The administration of the vignettes followed the original model. Respondents were asked to read an instruction card which was reinforced by oral directions from the interviewer (S.F.). They were told to rate the seriousness of each incident on a scale from 1 (least serious) to 9 (most serious). To achieve the maximum independence between each rating, the vignettes were presented singly on cards which had been shuffled into random order before each interview.

The rating process yielded a single score for each vignette which indicated both the strength and the direction of the respondent's perception. This method has the advantage of enabling particular incidents to be isolated and rated systematically by all respondents. It becomes possible to compare a range of occurrences which would be impracticable to achieve by direct observation of their work with families and children. The response rate is higher than a postal survey could obtain, and the use of a closed method to yield a single score facilitates analysis. Moreover, the adoption of an established instrument allows one to benefit from the original testing for reliability (Giovannoni and Becerra, 1979, p. 106).

However, there are certain problems about the validity of the technique. There is no necessary relationship between the definitions of mistreatment elicited by the vignettes and the actual behaviour of respondents. On the other hand, one could reasonably infer that this method does at least tap part of the general frame of reference within which decisions are made about specific cases. Unsolicited remarks by respondents confirmed that they were using their own experience in the judgements, and most seemed to have had some cases which were remarkably similar to those described in the vignettes. Some respondents did find difficulty in performing the exercise on the limited information given. Vignette 11 caused particular problems because the severity of the congenital heart defect was unspecified and it was clear that a number of respondents would have regarded that as a factor influencing their own concern. As one health visitor pointed out, though, when a family moves into a new area the minimal information represented by the vignettes is frequently all that a health visitor would have available to determine her priority for visiting. The same may well be true for intake social workers.

The respondents

The vignettes were pre-tested with five social work students, to familiarize the interviewer with the technique and to estimate the time required, which varied between 15 and 20 minutes. They were then administered to a sample of 20 social workers and 20 health visitors, all of whom were working in a prosperous university town in southern England. Although the numbers are relatively small, certain extrinsic sources of variation were removed. Both groups could rate the vignettes out of their experience working with the same

Table 9.1 Vignettes and ratings by social workers and health visitors

Vignette	Rating			
	Social workers		Health visitors	
	Mean	Standard deviation	Mean	Standard deviation
Sexual abuse				
1. On one occasion the parent and child engaged in mutual masturbation.	6.80	2.37	6.75	1.55
2. The parent repeatedly showed the child pornographic pictures. The child suffers recurring nightmares.	7.00	2.00	7.10	1.62
Physical abuse				
3. The parent burned the child on the buttocks and the chest with a cigarette. The child has second-degree burns.	8.80	0.41	8.80	0.41
4. The parents usually punish their child by spanking him with a leather strap, leaving red marks on his skin.	7.20	1.58	7.25	1.12
Emotional mistreatment				
5. The parents dress their son in girls' clothing, sometimes putting make-up on him. The child fights with other children.	6.30	1.81	6.25	1.68
6. A child has severe behaviour problems. The parents have allowed the child to undergo treatment but refuse to cooperate themselves.	5.50	1.36	5.50	1.96
Nutritional neglect				
7. The parents feed only milk to their child. The child has an iron deficiency.	5.85	2.21	4.90	2.36
8. The parents always insist that their child clean his plate, which they keep full of food. Doctors have warned that the child's health will suffer if he continues to eat so much.	4.40	1.27	4.80	2.02
Medical neglect				
9. The parents ignored the fact that their child was obviously ill, crying constantly and not eating. When they finally brought the child to a hospital he was found to be seriously dehydrated.	7.20	1.32	7.50	1.57

#	Item				
10.	The parents ignored their child's complaints of an ear-ache and chronic ear drainage. The child was found to have a serious ear infection and damage to the inner ear.	6.50	1.61	5.85	1.79
11.	The parents have repeatedly failed to keep medical appointments for their child. The child has a congenital heart defect.	5.95	1.76	6.15	1.73
12.	The parents have not taken their child to a dentist. The child has difficulty eating.	3.45	1.39	3.85	1.87

Supervision

#	Item				
13.	On one occasion the parents left their child alone all night.	6.30	1.66	7.25	1.97

Alcohol/drugs

#	Item				
14.	A parent experimented with cocaine while alone taking care of the child. The child swallowed a small box of laxatives.	6.95	1.70	7.15	1.42

Cleanliness

#	Item				
15.	The parents usually leave their child on a filthy, sodden mattress. The child has infected sores on his body.	7.55	1.19	7.60	1.05
16.	The parents do not wash their child's hair nor bathe the child for weeks at a time. He has impetigo in several places.	4.65	2.21	4.90	2.07

Parental sexual mores

#	Item				
17.	A divorced mother who has custody of her child brings home different men often. Her child knows about her sexual relations.	4.55	1.67	4.75	2.02

Clothing

#	Item				
18.	The parents always let their child run around the house and garden with out any clothes on. The child had a bad cold.	3.65	1.69	3.80	2.04

Housing

#	Item				
19.	The parents live with their child in an old house. Two windows in the living room where the child plays have been broken for some time and the glass has very jagged edges. The child cut his hand on the jagged edges, requiring three stitches.	5.40	2.04	5.75	1.97
20.	The parents live with their child in a small rented house. No-one ever cleans up. Decaying refuse, rats and cockroaches are everywhere.	5.65	1.60	6.45	1.57

population and under the same Area Review Committee procedural guide. The health visitors were selected, with their consent, by the Assistant Director of Nursing Services as a representative cross-section of her staff. The social workers were volunteers from the relevant area teams. Interviews were generally held in the respondents' offices.

Details about age, sex, child-rearing experience and data of professional qualification were collected. The social workers were younger (mean age 36.4 years against 40.8 years), more likely to be male (20 per cent against none) and to have child-rearing experience (55 per cent against 40 per cent). None of these showed any significant association with the ratings.

Results

The mean score and standard deviation for each vignette are shown in Table 9.1. The t-test was used to look for significant differences between the two groups. None were found, with the exception of V13 (the child being left alone all night on one occasion) which the health visitors scored somewhat more highly.

The health visitors and social workers were in clear agreement about the *relative* seriousness of the incidents described. When their ratings were compared on a ranking basis, i.e. considered high or low in relationship to the other items, the results also showed a great deal of similarity (Table 9.2). Both groups agreed as to the four most serious incidents: the parent burned the child on the buttocks and the chest with a cigarette leaving second-degree burns (V3); the parents usually leave their child on a filthy, sodden mattress and the child has infected sores on his body (V15); the parents usually punish their child by spanking him with a leather strap leaving red marks on the child's skin (V4); and the parents ignored the fact that their child was obviously ill, crying constantly and not eating. When they finally brought the child into hospital he was found to be seriously dehydrated (V9). So both vignettes concerned with physical abuse (V3 and V4) were rated seriously by the professionals despite what might have been regarded as a borderline between punishment and abuse in (V4). It is also interesting to note that the professionals appeared to differentiate between two similar incidents regarding cleanliness (V15 and V16), rating the former as very serious and the latter as one of the least serious. In fact both groups agreed about which incidents they considered least serious; V8, V12, V16, V17, V18. These generally low scores suggest that for most respondents there was doubt about whether these incidents/situations in fact constituted mistreatment.

Discussion

The striking features of these data is the lack of differences between health visitors' and social workers' perceptions of potential child care problems. Although there were certain background differences these did not produce associated differences in the interpretation of the vignettes. For this group

Table 9.2 Ranking of vignettes according to seriousness rating

Social workers		Health visitors	
Vignette no.	Mean	Vignette no.	Mean
3	8.8	3	8.8
15	7.55	15	7.6
4	7.2	9	7.5
9	7.2	4	7.25
2	7.0	13	7.25
14	6.95	14	7.15
1	6.8	2	7.1
10	6.5	1	6.75
5	6.3	20	6.45
13	6.3	5	6.25
11	5.95	11	6.15
7	5.85	10	5.85
20	5.65	19	5.75
6	5.5	6	5.5
19	5.4	7	4.9
16	4.65	16	4.9
17	4.55	8	4.8
8	4.4	17	4.75
18	3.65	12	3.85
12	3.45	18	3.8

there are good grounds for talking of a common approach. One question which might be raised, however, is whether this is due to health visitors moving towards social workers or vice versa. In other words, are both groups close to a 'medical' pole or to a 'social' pole?

Some clues may be found by comparing the results from this study with the scores obtained by Giovannoni and Becerra for American paediatricians and social workers. This comparison must be treated with caution because of the differences in the two studies and in the institutional contexts of practice. What it reveals, however, is that health visitors and social workers are more like each other than they are like either of the American groups. At a significance level of $p < 0.05$, the health visitors differed from the paediatricians on 10 of the 20 vignettes (V1, V4, V7, V8, V11–V13, V16, V20); in all of these except V1 the health visitors viewed the incidents more severely. At the same significance level the British social workers differed from their American counterparts on nine vignettes (V1, V4, V6, V13–V15, V17–V20); in all of these the British social workers viewed the incidents less severely. These findings are consistent with an argument that the British occupations are occupying a common ground which has not been sharply demarcated by their previous training.

It must be stressed that this was a small study whose results cannot be treated as conclusive. Nevertheless, it does lead us to question certain well-established policy assumptions. One is the view that referral difficulties between health visitors and social workers derive from differences in their perception of problems and can be remedied by joint training in a shared approach. We may do better to consider the organizational barriers to effective teamwork and the ways in which they might be reduced. Of course, similar studies comparing other groups might yield evidence of differences which could profitably be discussed in the sort of multi-disciplinary training packages which have become popular: the point is to question their value if they only embrace social workers and health visitors.

More broadly, however, it does lead us to ask exactly what a nursing background is contributing to health visiting. A full answer would obviously involve a much bigger study over a greater range of topics. Even so, these findings should give some cause for reflection on the necessity of nurse training for health visiting. This is not to say health visiting could or should be collapsed into social work: there are good arguments why these functions should be separated. It may, however, be the case that a much broader pool of people could become satisfactory health visitors than is currently possible. Alternatively, perhaps we should be asking whether the clinical elements of health visiting should be enhanced, perhaps creating a community paediatric nurse practitioner, to make better use of the expensive prior training investment than may currently be the case.

All of these conclusions are, of course, highly tentative. However, we hope that the findings may be of sufficient interest to challenge others to further replications and extensions of this work.

Reference

Giovannoni, J. M. and Becerra, R. M. (1979). *Defining Child Abuse*. Collier-Macmillian, London.

## 10

Health and material deprivation in Plymouth

Pamela Abbott, Joyce Bernie, Geoff Payne and Roger Sapsford

Introduction

The aim of this chapter is to provide a summary of health inequalities in the Plymouth Health District (PHD). It is now well established that there is a relationship between material deprivation and health status and that inequalities in both exist even within small areas. This chapter explores in a relatively small area the relationship illustrated on a national scale by the Black Report. The overall findings are that areas of relatively extreme deprivation and poor health can be identified, almost as bad as the worst of the London wards described in other studies.

The Black Report's publication in 1980 had a significant impact on both politicians and the medical and medical–sociology disciplines. The working group's main finding was the apparent failure of post-war social welfare and economic policy significantly to reduce the difference in health experience between the most affluent and the most impoverished in our society. Except in the case of child health, the differential between occupational classes I and II on the Registrar General's scale (professional and managerial) and classes IV and V (semi- and unskilled manual workers) in terms of life expectancy had grown wider. Infant mortality rates for the more affluent in society had fallen steadily, while the death rate for the poorest had fallen only marginally, which meant that differences in adult mortality rate had actually worsened (Black Report 1980, p. 74). In the same period, the number of people in poverty had also increased – those in the lower social classes, obviously, being more likely to be in poverty.

Since the publication of the Black Report there has been an extensive effort by social scientists to investigate health inequalities, including a number of small-area studies. Researchers have looked at a number of potential associations between social and material deprivation indicators and health indicators – moving away from occupational or social class as the sole indicator of differences in lifestyle. A range of factors have been found to be associated with different levels of mortality and morbidity: occupational class, unemployment, income, car ownership, gender, race, age, marital status, area of residence, and so on (Black Report, 1980; Moser *et al.*, 1986; Wilkinson, 1986; Townsend *et al.*, 1986a,b; MacIntyre, 1986; Marsh and Channing, 1986; Whitehead, 1987). The small-area studies have consistently found an association between ill health and deprivation (Table 10.1) – Townsend *et al.* (1986a,b) arguing that deprivation measures are more highly associated with health deprivation than is social class.

Looking at unemployment, Moser *et al.* (1986) found that even after socio-economic distribution is taken into account, there remains an excess of ill health, and it is not due to health selection – in other words, it is not necessarily the people who were previously least healthy who become unemployed. The stress associated with unemployment could be implicated in raised suicide rates among the unemployed, and the level of mortality of women married to unemployed men is worse than for other married women. Moser *et al.* (1986) conclude that unemployment is associated with adverse effects on health. Wilkinson (1986) found that there was a statistically significant negative

Table 10.1   Deprivation and ill health: small-area analyses

Authors	Study	Findings
Carstairs (1981)	37 municipal wards in Glasgow and 23 in Edinburgh	Good evidence of greater mortality and morbidity in areas of greater deprivation (except for perinatal and infant deaths)
Fox *et al.* (1984)	36 clusters of wards in England and Wales	Pattern of low mortality in high-status clusters and high in low-status clusters. Longitudinal study
Thunhurst (1985)	29 wards in Sheffield	Clear correlation between 'areas of poverty' and mortality. For men, life expectancy was over 8 years more in the most affluent wards than in the least
Townsend *et al.* (1985)	28 wards in Bristol	Poor health significantly correlated with deprivation
Townsend *et al.* (1986a)	755 wards in London	Mortality rate of the most deprived wards nearly double that of the least deprived
Townsend *et al.* (1986b)	678 wards in Northern Region	Correspondence between ill health and deprivation extremely close. The strongest association between health and deprivation variables was with lack of car (proxy for low income)

association of health with changes of income, suggesting that small changes in the living standards of occupational class V families literally mean life or death to the babies born to them. Higher levels of mortality are associated with living in rented accommodation and with not having access to a car. Car ownership, as an indicator of material deprivation, was found by Townsend *et al.* (1986a) to be highly correlated with poor health status as measured by their Health Index (which included measures of mortality, morbidity and child development).

The Black Report cited 'material deprivation' as a major factor in explaining health inequalities. Its authors also highlighted the need for more detailed information to augment present understanding, if any improvement in health status was to be achieved. It is also now apparent that great inequality in health can exist between small areas in the same region. The advantage of working at a regional or Health District level is that those wards within larger geographical areas which experience relatively high levels of ill health can be identified. Townsend and his colleagues have developed a set of research methods which enables this type of research to be undertaken. Easily available statistical data, at ward level, can be extracted from the 1981 Census and OPCS birth/death data to construct a Health Index and a Material Deprivation Index which can then be compared. These developments have been used in this report to investigate the existence of health inequalities in the PHD and their relationship to material deprivation. Plymouth is chosen in the first instance because of local interest. However, the PHD is one of the largest in the country and contains a mix of areas from inner-city urban wards to very typically rural areas, both of which make it a relevant area for study. It is also located within a region which is relatively advantaged overall in terms both of material wealth and of health status, but (as we shall see) the gross regional statistics mask a very considerable degree of variation.

The Plymouth Health District

Plymouth Health is one of several Districts within the South-West Health Region. The region as a whole is one of the most advantaged in Great Britain in terms of mortality data, having the second lowest standardized death rate for men, the third lowest for single women and the lowest for married women. (However, one should remember that there are variations in mortality based on social class – men in social classes IV and V have a standardized mortality ratio 56 per cent higher than men in social classes I and II – see Table 10.2). Compared to the national experience the South West is relatively healthy, having some of the lowest mortality rates in the country (Deacon, 1987, p. 10).

The total population served by the PHD is 387 384, of whom 297 985 live in urban areas and 89 399 in wholly rural areas – 77% and 23% respectively (1981 Census data). The majority of the population live within the twenty Plymouth City wards. While all twenty of the wards in the Plymouth City

Table 10.2 Standardized Mortality Ratio (all causes) in the South-West region, by occupational class, 1979–80 and 1982–3 (source: OPCS, 1986)

Class	Men	Women
I and II	69	70
IV and V	108	96
IV and V as Percentage of I and II	156	137

Note: The national average SMR is 100. Women are classified here on own occupation, or on husband's if not employed.

District are classified as urban, in the less remote rural areas less than half the population live in exclusively urban wards, and in North Cornwall only one fifth. While Plymouth City itself has the lowest pensioner population as a proportion of the total for the district, and South Hams (at almost 20 per cent) the highest percentage of residents over 65 years of age, the population of the PHD as a whole is characterized by a significant proportion of elderly people. The age-adjusted standardized mortality rates (SMRs) for the PHD (i.e. making allowance for demographic differences in the age distribution but calculating a separate index for each sex) are 101.5 for men and 95.9 for women; the overall national SMR is of course 100. Unemployment for the PHD area as a whole was slightly lower than the UK average at the time of the 1981 Census.

The PHD in fact covers a large geographical area surrounding the city of Plymouth – from Looe (Cornwall) in the West to Kingsbridge on the South Devon coast east of Plymouth, and as far north as Launceston (North Cornwall) and Tavistock (West Devon). The five local authority districts served by the PHD are Plymouth City, South Hams, West Devon, Caradon and North Cornwall. Within the PHD there is a diversity of social and economic environments. Plymouth City is the industrial service centre for the immediate locality, with employment prospects closely tied to the naval dockyards, light industry and the service sector. The city is surrounded by less remote rural areas – South Hams, West Devon and Caradon – through which medium-sized towns are scattered. These areas were characterized by a very low rate of unemployment at the time of the 1981 Census – less than two-thirds of the national rate. Finally, on the periphery of the PHD service area is North Cornwall, a remote rural area containing a few small market towns.

The following descriptions of each of the districts has been put together from the OPCS publication by John Craig, *Studies on Medical and Population Subjects* No. 48, which classifies towns and districts into 'families' by their points of similarity and difference in demographic and industrial terms; the description of the various criteria are all relative to the distributions of these criteria in Great Britain as a whole. Plymouth City is classified under family '4B (19)', a less industrial regional centre; the most typical representative of this family in Craig's study is Bristol. The demographic structure of Plymouth shows an excess of young people in the 15–24 age-group and of people of pensionable age. There are more one-person (non-pensioner) households and a slightly higher migrant population, which reflects the impact of the Forces and the Polytechnic on the city. Housing tenure figures are the same as the UK average in terms of owner–occupation, local authority and unfurnished letting, but there is an excess of furnished accommodation and accommodation with shared amenities. Overcrowding is slightly lower than the national figure. Use of public transport to work is marginally lower than the national average, as is ownership of two or more cars. In terms of social class, there are marginally more non-manual and unskilled heads of household and fewer professional, managerial, skilled and semi-skilled workers. Manufacturing and the service industries provide the majority of the employment opportunities.

South Hams, Caradon and West Devon fall into the '2a (9)' category. Typically these districts are characterized by a population which is middle-aged to elderly. These are fewer large families or one-person (non-pensioner) households. There is an excess of owner–occupation and less local authority housing than the national average. Employment is dominated by the service sector and agriculture. There are more professional/managerial and non-manual employees and fewer manual heads of household. Households owning two cars or more are frequent, 14.5 times the UK average; use of public transport for journey to work is low, only a third of the national figure.

North Cornwall is the only remote rural area in the PHD, classified under 'family 2a (8)'. The population tends to be elderly. Housing tenure patterns are slightly different from the other rural areas in that there is an excess of private unfurnished lettings and less local authority housing; owner occupation is at about the UK mean. There are fewer non-manual and unskilled but more skilled manual heads of household than the UK norm. Use of public transport to work is very rare, and there is a slightly higher than average ownership of two or more cars. Occupational opportunities are dominated by agriculture – at five times the national average – with less than average opportunities in manufacturing and service industries.

Measuring deprivation in the Plymouth Health District

In order to examine the relationship between deprivation and health status in the PHD and to locate the areas with poor health status, we have used the methods developed by Townsend *et al.* (1985, 1986a,b) to study other areas of England. This involved the construction of a Deprivation Index and a Health Status Index as two composites of various indicators, and a comparison of the two using multiple regression techniques. In discussing the results of the analysis we frequently highlight the highest and lowest quintile (the highest fifth of the wards and the lowest fifth) on a given measure. This enables us to see clearly which are the highest and lowest 17 wards on any given indicator, out of the total of 85. However, this is only a rough guide to distribution or relationship. For the key deprivation indicators we also look at the deviation from the 'normal curve' – the distribution which would be expected if the behaviours and experiences of individuals were randomly distributed with respect to the indicators. The indicators are often expressed as 'z-scores' – in statistical terms, they have been 'normalized' – so that a high positive score means that a ward is substantially more deprived than the average in the PHD, for example, and a high negative score means that it is substantially less deprived.

A minor refinement of our method over Townsend's is that we have gone through a double normalization process in order to relate our scores directly to what would be the expected distribution if traits were randomly distributed (the Normal Curve). This enables us not only to pick out *which* wards are at the extremes of the distribution, but to say *by how much* they deviate. If traits were randomly distributed, we might expect 95 per cent of scores (perhaps all but 3 or 4 of the 85 wards of the PHD) to lie between scores of about plus or minus 2.0, and 99 per cent (effectively, all) to lie between scores of about plus or minus 2.5. Thus scores more extreme than this are cause for concern – not just random deviations, but of sufficient extremity to suggest strongly an underlying 'cause'.

It must be stressed that the composite Deprivation and Health Indices discussed in this report are 'normed' for the PHD – that is, they measure extremity of deviation from the PHD average, not from some absolute or national average. They permit comparison within the PHD but cannot be compared with indices developed for other areas and calculated as deviations from those areas averages. What they enable us to do is to look at the distribution of the wards in the PHD, to see which are around the average on both indices, which are extreme (and how extreme) on either index, and the extent to which the two indices correlate (pick out the same wards as being extreme or average).

The basic data used to construct the Deprivation Index came from the 1981 Census Small Area Statistics. These gave a range of measures for each ward of the PHD. All 'deprivation' variables were converted to z-scores ('normalized') for the purpose of constructing the Deprivation Index. This procedure has the advantages that it irons out differences in units of measurement and provides an interpretable spread of figures. The *disadvantage* is that all variables are expressed relative to the PHD norm. We *can* compare z-scores between wards in the PHD, but we *cannot* compare z-scores for Plymouth with z-scores for some other part of the country, because the other scores will be expressed as deviations from some different average value. (However, we *can* make comparisons with other areas on each of the single indicators which have gone to make up the composite Indices. A comparison of the worst and best wards in Plymouth with London boroughs on the single variables used to construct the Deprivation Index suggests that the worst ward in Plymouth is not much less deprived than the worst wards in London. At the other end of the scale, the best wards in London seem to be a great deal more advantaged than the best wards in the PHD. The former finding is surprising, given that there are many more wards in London than in the PHD and thus we would expect a wider range by chance alone.)

The research reviews (e.g. Wilkinson 1986; Whitehead, 1987) illustrate the vast range of deprivation indicators available as tools for this kind of research. Townsend *et al.* have suggested that the available indicators can be divided into two groups: indicators of *states* of deprivation and indicators of the *victims* of deprivation. States of deprivation imply a relative lack of material resources, which in turn mitigates against 'engagement in the normal activities of individuals in the wider society' (LeGrand and Robinson, 1985, p. 219). Material deprivations comprise 'lack of goods, services, resources, amenities and physical environment' (Townsend *et al.* 1986a, p. 49). Some indicators of material deprivation are direct measures of this aspect of the concept – for example income; those living solely on state benefits, for example, cannot by any stretch of the imagination be described as materially privileged. Other indicators are more indirect and may be assumed to reflect lack of income – housing tenure (not owner–occupier), for example.

Indicators of the victims of deprivation are in essence variables identifying groups of people as *at risk* of experiencing material deprivation. Single-parent families, being elderly and living alone, being a household whose head is in social class IV or V, being an ethnic minority household, are all variables of this type. They are not direct measures of deprivation – not all households in these categories are deprived – but statistically the probability of deprivation is greater if one is in such a category, so they indicate risk of deprivation. The danger of using these social categories as indicators of deprivation, Townsend *et al.* argue, is that one may be led into the assumption that being elderly, for instance, is in itself indicative of deprivation. Clearly there are examples of elderly people who live alone and are materially privileged relative to their peers. Discovering proportions of the population within wards who represent these social categories presumed to be 'at risk' of material deprivation does not necessarily give us the proportion actually suffering material deprivation. Townsend *et al.* (1986b) argue that these social categories are more indicative of *social* deprivation – 'non-participation in roles, relationships, customs, functions, rights and responsibilities implied by membership of society' (p. 49). As far as this study is concerned, the main objective is to investigate the existence of a specific relationship between health experience and material deprivation. It is beyond its scope to try to uncover the intricate social conditions and interactions associated with an individual's health experience and health-promoting behaviour. We have therefore followed Townsend *et al.* (1986a,b) in using only 'state of deprivation' variables in constructing our Deprivation Index. However, it is important to keep in mind that specific groups such as the elderly do suffer higher levels of morbidity than the rest of the population, independently of any effect of material deprivation, and may require a disproportionate share of health resources.

As already indicated, the PHD is made up of both urban and rural wards. There is a body of literature which contests the validity for rural areas of the indicators used to uncover urban deprivation (e.g. Cullingford and

Openshaw, 1982; Phillips and Williams, 1984; Fearn, 1987). Studies which rely on social area analysis are particularly vulnerable to underrating rural deprivation, it is suggested. Indeed, Townsend *et al.* constructed their new material deprivation index for use in the Northern Regional Health Authority because it was felt that previous deprivation indices tended disproportionately to 'favour' circumstances prevalent in inner cities.

There are, however, practical constraints on the use of the data derived from Census Small Area Statistics which restrict their usefulness for rural wards. First, rural wards have small populations; and the small area statistics are derived from a ten per cent sample of the Census, not the full data set. Thus they may sometimes be unrepresentative of the ward population as a whole. Secondly, ward boundaries are arbitrary and do not necessarily indicate discrete communities or homogeneous areas. Rural wards which cover large geographical areas could be described as microcosms of UK society, a mixture of well-to-do and poor; rural wards tend to be much more heterogeneous than urban wards (Cullingford and Openshaw, 1982, p. 412). This may influence the values of the deprivation indicators to the extent that the apparent level of deprivation shown overall in a ward may mask or even emphasize and exaggerate the actual level of localized instances of material deprivation within it.

Any study which compares *areas* and draws conclusions from them about *people* is at risk of committing the 'ecological fallacy', and the current study is no exception. If an area shows a high level of deprivation, it does not necessarily follow that all the people in that area are deprived. Wards can be large enough that even the 'deprived' ones contain pockets of middle-class housing and the 'non-deprived' ones have some areas of poverty and deprivation. (We could have based our analysis on smaller areas – census enumeration districts, say – but the same problem would still persist to some extent. We should also have encountered the problem that the Small Area Statistics are deliberately modified where very small units of population are concerned, by the addition or subtraction of a random factor, in order to protect confidentiality.) An 'average' area could be average because it contains all 'average' people, or because it is made up of equal numbers from each extreme. Thus we cannot say absolutely that identifying a deprived area or an area of poor health is the same as identifying the people / households who are deprived or in poor health. Where health and deprivation correlate we cannot even say absolutely that it is the deprived people who have poor health, though this seems extremely likely. All we can assert with confidence is that if areas of high deprivation are also areas of poor health, then 'targeting' these areas in terms of resource provision should mean putting resources within the reach of a larger than average number of those who most need them.

Having noted these reasons for being cautious in interpretation of the data, we shall now consider possible deprivation indicators which have been used in previous research and their distribution in Plymouth, one at a time, and finally the construction of a single overall Index of Deprivation.

Social class

In previous research, social class has been used as a proxy indicator of disadvantage. In the PHD there are marked differences by area in the distribution of households whose heads are recorded as being in the lowest or the highest social classes. Only one ward had more than 40 per cent of households in social classes IV or V (semi- and un-skilled manual labour), but there are five wards with between 30 and 40 per cent, the PHD average being 17.85 per cent. There are many more wards with a marked concentration of social classes I and II (professional and managerial). This suggests that there are more advantaged than disadvantaged areas in the PHD. There are problems, however, in using household social class as a sole indicator of deprivation. Some we have discussed above. Another is that the wide variation in salaries/ wages between occupations within the same social class means that social class is not necessarily a good indicator of income differentials. There is also the fact that household social class is based on the occupation of the 'head of household' and does not take account of the occupations of other members of the household. The increased proportion of wives in paid employment and making an economic contribution to the household means that households in the same social class can have widely differing levels of income; in 1989 six out of every ten mothers with children younger than ten were in paid employment (OPCS, 1990).

Single-parent households

Lone parents and their children are likely to be materially and socially deprived. Single-parent households are also concentrated in particular areas within the PHD. Only one ward outside of Plymouth City has 8 per cent or more of single-parent households, but three wards within the City boundaries have this concentration.

Lone-pensioner households

These are more widely distributed in the PHD – which would be expected, given that the area is a retirement one. While lone pensioners may be socially deprived, they are not necessarily materially deprived. However, elderly people, and especially those living alone, are likely to make heavy demands on the health services. Sixteen wards in the PHD have over 17 per cent of lone-pensioner households.

Children under five years of age

Households with young children are more concentrated in the Plymouth City area than outside it. Only three wards, and all in the City, have over 25 per cent of households with children under five years of age. There are twelve wards that have between 20 and 25 per cent of such households. While there is no necessary correlation between deprivation and proportion of households with young children, such households present an increased demand for health services.

Lack of basic amenities

The vast majority of households in the PHD have the use of an inside bathroom and/or w.c. Only ten wards have more than three per cent of households without these basic amenities. While lack of basic amenities is clearly an indicator of deprivation and has been taken as such in previous studies, there are problems in its use. Some of the otherwise most deprived households live in council accommodation, which does *not* lack these basic amenities. Similarly, it is general practice to assume that living with shared amenities – not having self-contained accommodation – is an indicator of deprivation. However, in a town such as Plymouth with a large student population there are problems in accepting this at face value.

Households without a car

As would be expected, households without a car are more concentrated in urban areas and specifically in Plymouth City. Of the eleven wards where more than 40 per cent of households do not have the use of a car, only one is *not* within the Plymouth City boundaries. The PHD average is 26.5 per cent of households without a car.

Overcrowded households

Only two wards in the PHD have seven per cent or more of households that are recorded as overcrowded (with more than one person per room in the accommodation), both within Plymouth City.

Housing Tenure

Five wards have a high proportion of households living in rented accommodation. Thirteen wards have less than 25 per cent of households in rented accommodation. The PHD average is 37 per cent of households in property which they do not own.

Unemployment

Unemployment is highly concentrated by area. Only two wards have more than 18 per cent of the population of working age unemployed – St Peter's and Lydford. On the whole, higher levels of unemployment are to be found in the Plymouth City area than in the areas outside the city. However, six wards in the areas outside the city show high levels of unemployment, while six city wards show relatively low levels. The PHD average is 9.5 per cent. (One should note, however, that these data are derived from the 1981 Census and may have been changed by subsequent events).

The Deprivation Index

Four indicators from the 1981 Census have been used to construct an overall index of deprivation, using the technique of converting the raw figures to z-scores, adding these together and then renormalizing to give a new z-score

1. *Unemployment*: the percentage of economically active residents aged 16 to 59 or 64 (according to gender) who are unemployed.
2. *Car ownership*: the percentage of private households without the use of a car.
3. *Home ownership*: the percentage of private households which are *not* owner-occupied.
4. *Overcrowding*: the percentage of private households with more than one person per room.

Unemployment not only reflects individual income and lack of access to material resources; it also reflects community deprivation. High levels of unemployment within a small population affect aspects of the local economy – for example, in terms of the type of retail outlet available, particularly food outlets (Hamilton-Cole and Lang, 1986) – which in turn may affect community health status within these areas. Townsend *et al.* (1986b) state that 'unemployment is an indicator which is acknowledged to be very wide in scope as well as reliable'. The lack of car ownership is thought to be the best surrogate for current income levels. (In an area of mixed urban and rural wards its quality as an indicator is more questionable. It seems likely that car ownership in rural wards would, of necessity, remain at quite high levels relative to that of urban wards where public transport is available. Even those who are on low incomes would strive to maintain their mobility in rural areas through car possession. Centralization of services has meant that car ownership is more essential for families living in outlying villages – see Fearn, 1987, p. 264.) Though there are high levels of car ownership in the UK – 79 per cent in rural areas and 59 per cent in urban ones, according to the 1981 Census – this does not necessarily indicate greater access to resources in rural wards. It could be further argued that the 21 per cent of rural households not owning a car suffer significant isolation and disadvantage in access to health services centralized in Plymouth, relative to their urban counterparts (see again, Fearn, 1987). To assess the contribution of car ownership to the overall index of material deprivation, separate regression analyses have been carried out for urban and rural wards in the PHD.

Not owning one's own house is an indicator of lack of wealth as well as lack of income. Though in some individual cases lack of income may not be the primary reason for renting, nonetheless the level of owner-occupation is widely accepted as a valid indicator of access to moderate income and long-term wealth.

Overcrowding is used to reflect poor housing conditions and is inclined to balance the effects of owner-occupation; adequately large housing has been made more available to people of more modest income in recent years in the rented sector. Those who are both in rented accommodation and over-crowded are therefore doubly and unusually deprived.

When these four indicators are combined to form an overall Deprivation Index, they are found to be relatively highly intercorrelated (Table 10.3) – wards high on one variable tend to be high on the others. An overall measure of their average correlation, Cronbach's alpha, indicates that the scale is relatively unidimensional (measuring a single underlying variable) by its reasonably high value of 0.81. An examination of the Deprivation Index scores for the wards in the PHD indicates that some are very materially deprived, while others show a fair degree of material advantage. Given that the scores are normalized, a score of zero indicates the exact average for the PHD; less than zero (a minus score) indicates a better than average 'material state', and greater than zero (a plus score) indicates some degree of material disadvantage. What we find is that the distribution is heavily skewed. If we take scores between plus and minus 1 (the range in which we would expect about two-thirds of the wards to fall) as the 'average range', we find that it includes 68 of the 85 PHD wards – around the expected number. A further seven wards score more extremely in a negative direction – they are substantially less deprived than the average. These comprise three Plymouth City wards, two in South Hams and two in West Devon. At the other end of the distribution we have ten wards which show substantial material deprivation on this Index – scores of more than + 1. Five of them are in the range from + 1 to + 2 – four in Plymouth City and one in Caradon. The others score more extremely disadvantaged than the highest-scoring 'advantaged' ward scores at the other end of the distribution; they are all in Plymouth City. The two most extreme, St Peter's and Ham, have scores respectively of 4.16 and 3.32 – values more extreme than one would ever expect in a random sample of this size.

A fair summary of the distribution is that the PHD has some wards which are much less deprived than others, but the difference is not dramatic. On the other hand, it would appear that the PHD has some wards which are very deprived indeed – a long 'tail' of Deprivation Index scores of increasingly extreme size. This picture is born out by comparison of the more extreme PHD wards (in both directions) with wards in London given; the PHD has nothing as extreme as the best of the London wards, but St Peter's ranks well up (or rather, down) with the worst of the London wards. Maps 1 and 3 illustrate,

Table 10.3   Correlations of the elements (in per cent) of a Deprivation Index

Element	Unemployed	No car	Not owner–occupier	Overcrowded
Unemployed	1.00			
No car	0.59	1.00		
Not owner–occupier	0.48	0.53	1.00	
Overcrowded	0.49	0.47	0.55	1.00

respectively, the best and the worst quintile on the Deprivation Index – the least and the most deprived fifth of wards.

It is clear from this analysis that the deprivation in the PHD is for the most part clustered in the inner city of Plymouth (though there are pockets of rural deprivation). Indeed, it is also evident that the separate indicators of deprivation cluster together in urban wards to a much greater extent than in rural ones. In other words, urban wards with a high proportion of unemployed persons as compared with the Plymouth mean also tend to have a high proportion of households with no car, of households living in accommodation they do not own, and of overcrowded housing. For rural wards, however, there is less relationship between the various indicators (Table 10.4). A closer inspection of the correlation matrix suggests that being unemployed and not owning a car may be correlated, but they share not much more than 14 per cent of their variance; the same variables share over 77 per cent of their variance in the analysis of urban wards. This seems to indicate, as suggested earlier, that people will strive to maintain a car in rural areas at much lower levels of income than in urban ones.

To sum up, the PHD area's separate indicators of deprivation tend to be clustered in the urban wards but not in the rural wards. This suggests that it is possible to determine deprived areas (wards) in urban areas – areas where a high proportion of the population are deprived relative to the rest of the PHD. It is not possible to do this well for the rural areas using the same indicators.

An analysis of a wider range of deprivation indicators, including some not chosen for inclusion in the Index constructed for this study, indicates that all of them are highly intercorrelated (Table 10.5). Using stepwise multiple correlation to test the Index against other possible combinations of indicators showed that other combinations would have worked equally as well as the combination used to make up the Deprivation Index. (Stepwise multiple correlation is a technique in which the best predictor is taken as a baseline, the next best is added to it (allowing for overlap between the two), then the next, and so on until the improvement in prediction from adding another variable

Table 10.4 Correlations of the Deprivation Index items (in per cent) for the PHD

Ward	Unemployed	Without use of a car	Not owner– occupier	Overcrowded
Urban wards (*n* = 34)				
unemployed	1.00			
without use of a car	0.88	1.00		
not owner–occupier	0.76	0.74	1.00	
overcrowded	0.68	0.59	0.66	1.00
Rural wards (*n* = 51)				
unemployed	1.00			
without use of a car	0.39	1.00		
not owner–occupier	0.02	0.04	1.00	
overcrowded	0.10	0.04	0.27	1.00

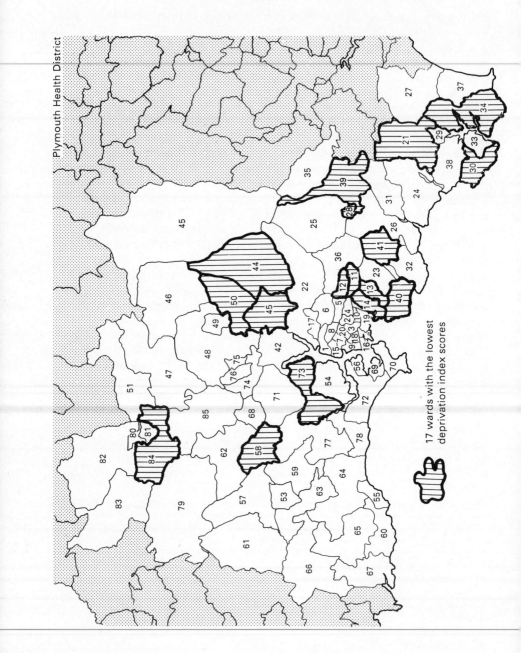

Plymouth Health District

17 wards with the lowest deprivation index scores

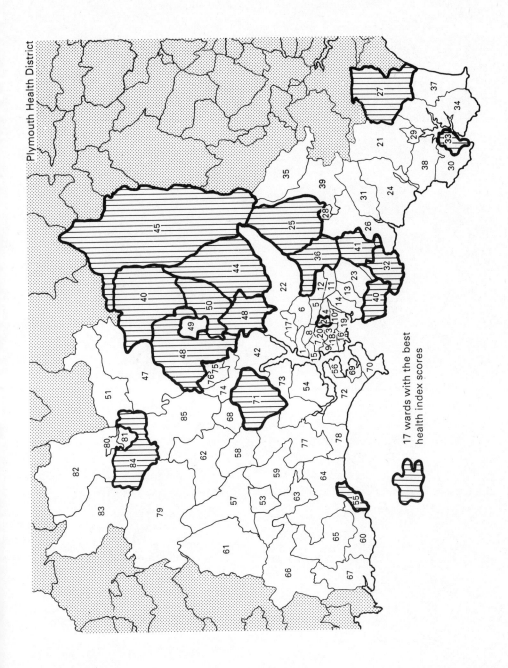

Plymouth Health District

17 wards with the best
health index scores

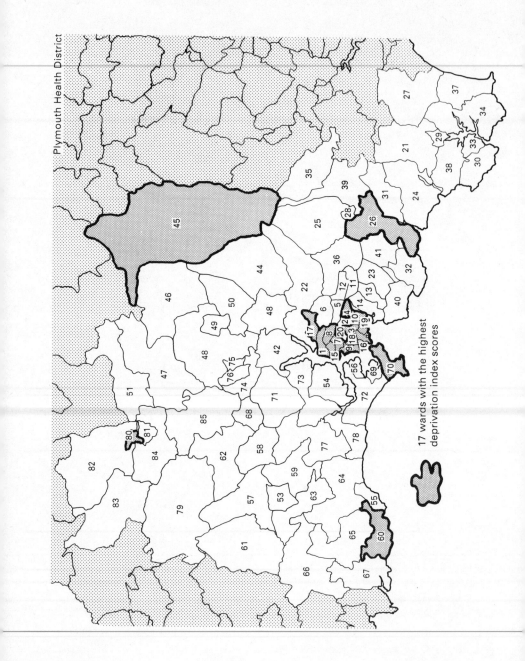

Plymouth Health District

17 wards with the highest deprivation index scores

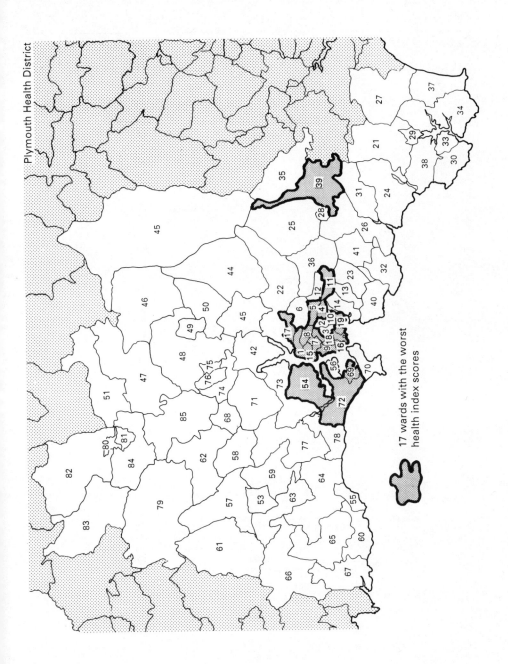

Plymouth Health District

17 wards with the worst health index scores

KEY TO MAPS

District	Ward Name	Type	Key
Plymouth City	Budshead	U	1
	Compton	U	2
	Drake	U	3
	Efford	U	4
	Eggbuckland	U	5
	Estover	U	6
	Ham	U	7
	Honicknowle	U	8
	Keyham	U	9
	Mount Gould	U	10
	Plympton Erle	U	11
	Plympton St Mary	U	12
	Plymstock Dunstone	U	13
	Plymstock Radford	U	14
	St Budeaux	U	15
	St Peter's	U	16
	Southway	U	17
	Stoke	U	18
	Sutton	U	19
	Trelawney	U	20
South Hams	Avonleigh	R	21
	Bickleigh	R	22
	Brixton	R	23
	Charterlands	R	24
	Cornwood	R	25
	Erne Valley	R	26
	Garabrook	R	27
	Ivybridge	U	28
	Kingsbridge	U	29
	Marlborough	R	30
	Modbury	R	31
	Newton & Noss	R	32
	Salcombe	U	33
	Saltstone	R	34
	S. Brent	U	35
	Sparkwell	R	36
	Stokenham	R	37
	Thurleston	R	38
	Ugborough	R	39
	Wembury	R	40
	Yealmpton	U	41
West Devon	Bere Ferrers	R	42
	Buckland Monachorum	R	43
	Burrator	R	44

District	Ward Name	Type	Key
	Lydford	R	45
	Mary Tavy	R	46
	Milton Ford	R	47
	Tamarside	R	48
	Tavistock N.	U	49
	Tavistock S.	U	50
	Thrushel	R	51
	Walkham	R	52
Caradon	Liskeard	U	53
	Saltash	U	54
	Looe	R	55
	Torpoint	U	56
	St Cleer	R	57
	St Ive	R	58
	Menheniot	R	59
	Lansallas	R	60
	St Neot	R	61
	Lyner	R	62
	Dobwalls	R	63
	Morval	R	64
	Trelawny	R	65
	Lanteglos	R	66
	St Veep	R	67
	Callington	U	68
	Millbrook	U	69
	Maker with Rame	R	70
	St Dominic	R	71
	Sheviock	R	72
	Landrake	R	73
	Calstock	R	74
	Chilworthy	R	75
	Gunnislake	R	76
	St Germans	R	77
	Downderry	R	78
North Cornwall	Altarnun	R	79
	Launceston N.	U	80
	Launceston S.	U	81
	N. Petherwine Ottery	R	82
		R	83
	S. Petherwin	R	84
	Stoke-climsland	R	85

U = urban; R = rural.

Table 10.5 Intercorrelation of possible deprivation indicators in the PHD

Indicator	A	B	C	D	E	F	G	H
A	1.00							
B	0.80	1.00						
C	0.81	0.59	1.00					
D	0.80	0.48	0.53	1.00				
E	0.78	0.49	0.47	0.55	1.00			
F	0.67	0.46	0.53	0.56	0.57	1.00		
G	0.25	0.36	0.46	0.00	−0.09	−0.08	1.00	
H	0.54	0.45	0.45	0.55	0.28	0.31	−0.67	1.00

Key: A = Deprivation Index; B = unemployed (%); C = without car (%); D = not owner–occupiers (%); E = overcrowded (%); F = single parents (%); G = lone pensioners (%); H = in classes IV/V (%).

ceases to be a significant one.) For example, a combination of incidence of single parenthood, proportion of lone-pensioner households and proportion of households headed by someone in social class IV or V yielded a multiple correlation of around 0.78 with the Deprivation Index and so shared around 61 per cent of its variance, and adding proportion of households headed by someone in social class I or II raised the proportion of shared variance to nearly 63 per cent. A plot of residuals – the unexplained variance left over – showed them to be more or less randomly scattered around the prediction line. Thus while we picked our indicators to cover particular kinds of deprivation, for good theoretical reasons, it would appear that almost any set of indicators would give as good an overall measure, as different types of deprivation are strongly clustered by area.

This conclusion holds only for urban areas, however, where the combination of indicators which we did not use shared over 80 per cent of variance with the Deprivation Index. In rural areas alone it shared only 16 per cent. This reinforces the argument that deprivation appears substantially less easy to identify in rural areas than in urban ones. It does not necessarily mean that deprivation is *not* geographically concentrated in particular rural areas, but it does indicate that this type of analysis *at ward level* does not identify such clusters of deprivation.

Health indicators for the PHD study

There is at present a limited range of available health data covering the whole population at the level of wards, which restricts the extent to which health status can be operationalized adequately. The measures used by Townsend *et al.* (1986b) to build a composite health index were Standardized Mortality Ratio (for both sexes under the age of 65, averaged over the three years 1981–3), proportion of residents in private households who described themselves as permanently sick or disabled (in the 1981 Census), and a measure of delayed development, the proportion of live births weighing below 2800 g, based on birth data for the three years 1982–4. (The Standardized Mortality Ratio is the ratio of actual deaths in an area to the number one would have expected if the area had the same age and gender composition as the country as a whole. The norm – the national death rate – is set at 100; higher figures mean that the area has more deaths than would be expected given the composition of its population, and lower figures that it has fewer deaths.) The justification presented by Townsend and his colleagues was that:

1. 'Premature death' SMRs provide the least ambiguous indicator of mortality at ward level.
2. Permanent sickness and disability data are not a measure of total level of morbidity in a ward, but they are the best available indicator from the Census of chronic health impairment.
3. Low birthweight is a measure not only of potential child development problems but also an indicator of maternal health.

The heath indicators used in the PHD study differ from Townsend's only for reasons of unavailability of data. The three measures used were:

1. *Mortality*: SMRs for both sexes aged 1–65, averaged over the five years 1982–6.
2. *Disablement*: the proportion of residents in private households classed as permanently sick or disabled in the 1981 Census.
3. *Infant mortality*: the rate of infant death (aged < 1 year) per thousand live births, averaged over the five years 1982–6.

The mortality statistics are averaged over five years to reduce the effect of yearly fluctuation, particularly in the wards with smaller populations. Infant mortality was substituted for low birthweight because the birthweight data were not readily available for all 85 wards in the PHD area. It has been used in previous studies (Black Report, 1980; Whitehead, 1987). While low birthweight is an indicator of maternal health and potential infant health, infant mortality is a reasonable measure of infant health – though a proportion of deaths will be the result of congenital conditions, birth trauma, etc. We were able to obtain low birthweight figures for Plymouth City itself, and these have been used in an alternative indicator.

These indicators were normalized – expressed as deviations from the PHD mean – added together and renormalized, in the same way as the indicators of material deprivation already discussed. The distribution in the PHD of the separate indicators and the composite Health Indices are discussed in the pages which follow.

Infant mortality

The infant mortality figures appear to reverse the trend for deprivation measures noted so far in this chapter. Few Plymouth City wards appear in the worst quintile. Wards with the best (i.e. lowest) infant mortality rate are mainly rural ones. The high number of wards with mortality rates of zero indicates one or more of three things: population artefact, low fertility rates or very good ante-natal and post-natal care. The 'population artefact' explanation – simply that very small wards have very few births and therefore little infant mortality – is discounted because the wards with the high populations (i.e. in Plymouth City) are not represented among the worst in significant numbers. The quality of care in the wards is discounted on the grounds that the districts represented in both extremes are similarly located; also, Plymouth City has the lion's share of ante-natal expertise, although non-attendance may have an effect here. The most plausible explanation is that the wards experiencing a high infant mortality rate have (a) high fertility rates (the more births, the greater the likelihood of deaths), combined with (b) poorer ante-natal provision (perhaps because of the remoteness of centrally based hospital provision from some wards). There is no significant difference between urban and rural areas.

Standardized Mortality Ratio

All of the wards with a low 'premature death' SMR lie outside the boundaries of Plymouth City, the majority being rural wards. However, both urban and rural wards are found among those with the worst, SMRs, with only six Plymouth City wards being included. The wide range of SMRs for wards will to a certain but unknown extent be an artefact of differences in ward population size. This problem is also probably applicable to measurements at district and urban/rural level. Thus in interpreting these data some caution must be exercised. Comparisons between Plymouth wards are probably the most valid.

Permanent sickness and disability

The proportion of the population reporting themselves permanently sick or disabled at the 1981 Census was relatively low. The highest proportion within a single ward of the PHD was 4 per cent (two wards), and the lowest 1 per cent (21 wards). Given the small variation in proportions there was no marked differences between urban and rural wards.

The composite health status indicators

Two composite indicators of health status were created. Health Index 1 replicates the index used by Townsend *et al.* (1985). In Health Index 2, low birthweight is replaced by infant mortality, as explained above. The correlation between the two indices for the Plymouth City wards is high, 0.89, indicating that they share 79 per cent of their variance. This suggests that Health Index 2 is a reasonable but not perfect proxy measure for Health Index 1.

The items which go to make up Health Index 1 are intercorrelated in the Plymouth City wards (Table 10.6). The distribution of scores on this measure for the Plymouth City wards is reasonably normal. The two wards with the

Table 10.6   Intercorrelation of items in Health Index 1

Item	Percentage permanently sick or disabled	Standardized Mortality Ratio	Low birthweight
Percentage permanently sick or disabled	1.00		
Standardized Mortality Ratio	0.50	1.00	
Low birthweight	0.58	0.68	1.00

highest scores are just over 1.75 standard deviations from the Plymouth City mean, while the ward with the lowest score lies about 1.5 standard deviations below it. In other words, there are no values as extreme as were found with the Deprivation Index; St Peter's has the worst score on Health Index 1, as it does on the Deprivation Index, but it does not stand out as much from the pack in respect of health as in respect of deprivation. However, one should remember that we are talking here only of deviations from the *Plymouth City* wards, data for other wards in the PHD being unavailable on Health Index 1, and there are only twenty of them. Given this small group size, one can fairly say that there is a substantial spread of values within Plymouth City from best to worst.

Health Index 2 uses infant mortality rates to replace low birthweight because of the unavailability of birthweight information for the wards outside Plymouth City. The items which go to make it up are again intercorrelated, but the correlations are low (Table 10.7). However, looking at the intercorrelations separately for urban and rural wards we find that the intercorrelations are higher for urban wards while there are no significant relationships in rural wards. As with the Deprivation Index, Health Index 2 was standardized, with a mean of zero for the PHD and the scores are expressed as standard deviations from the mean, with a positive score indicating greater ill health. The distribution is again skewed, with rather more extreme values for ill health than a random distribution would predict: we would not expect a score quite as high as St Peter's (3.32) in random distribution. However, the extremity is not as great as on the Deprivation Index. Of the seventeen highest-scoring wards all but three are urban wards, and of these all but one is in Plymouth City.

Of the seventeen wards with the lowest score on Health Index 2, only four

Table 10.7   Intercorrelation of items on Health Index 2

Item	Percentage permanently sick or disabled	Standardized Mortality Ratio	Infant mortality
Percentage permanently sick or disabled	1.00		
Standardized Mortality Ratio	0.28	1.00	
Infant mortality	0.12	0.30	1.00

are urban, and only one of these, Compton, in Plymouth City (two of the others being in South Hams and the third in West Devon). This illustrates that the rural areas experience the best health on the whole and the urban areas the poorest. The urban mean on Health Index 2 is 0.60, and the rural mean −0.40, a difference which is statistically significant. However, the distance from the overall mean for the most advantaged wards is not large − not nearly as large as the distance of the least advantaged wards from the mean. In other words, the variation in health status is not great and is about what one would expect by chance in a sample of this size, except at the worst end of the distribution where a handful of reasonably extreme scores are to be found.

The relationship between deprivation and health status indicators

The distribution of scores on both the Deprivation Index and Health Index 2 are skewed, with the most deprived wards on both indices being further from the mean than the most advantaged wards. The exceptionally disadvantaged wards are all in Plymouth City, the most disadvantaged ward on both Indices being St Peter's. (Maps 2 and 4 show the distribution respectively of the lowest and highest quintile of scores on Health Index 2.) Eight wards − St Peter's, Ham, Keyham, Sutton, St Budeaux, Honicknowle, Efford and Stoke − all in Plymouth City, are in the highest quintile for both deprivation and health scores, while six wards − Yealmpton, South Petherwine, Buckland Monachorum, Wembury, Tavistock South and Burrator − are in the lowest quintile for both. This comparison of extremes, however, underrates the degree of relationship between the Deprivation Index and Health Index 2. Cross-tabulating the two yields a positive correlation of 0.64, a reasonably high figure. A similar tabulation for Health Index 1, using only Plymouth City wards, indicates a similar degree of correlation.

When all 85 PHD wards were analysed together, the Deprivation Index came out a statistically significant predictor of Health Index 2, sharing 40 per cent of its variance. However, when we look at urban and rural wards separately we find that the Deprivation Index is a good predictor of Health Index 2 in urban areas − the two share 60 per cent of their variance − but that there is no significant relationship between the two for the rural wards. This indicates, as indeed we have suggested already, that is this method is good for identifying urban wards that are deprived and have poor health status, but that it is not as suitable for use in rural areas.

Lack of access to a car has been seen as a key predictor of health status in previous research (e.g. Townsend *et al.*, 1986b; Whitehead, 1987). This association holds for the 85 wards of the PHD when all are taken together. Using stepwise multiple regression to identify the order and importance of the individual predictive elements, car ownership enters the prediction first and explains about 48 per cent of the variance in Health Index 2 by itself. (However, it must be borne in mind (a) that there is a high level of intercorrelation between the variables, and (b) that the order of influence of variables is unstable, particularly when small samples are used. With a slightly larger or smaller geographical area, a different order of importance might have emerged.) Overcrowding entered the equation second, and the two variables together explained 51 per cent of variance. When the urban wards are considered by themselves, car ownership again enters the equation first, explaining about 57 per cent of variance, overcrowding raises the amount of variance explained to 63 per cent, and other indicators can raise it to about 70 per cent. By contrast, on the rural wards no significant prediction could be made at all.

As a further check on the validity of the Deprivation Index and its relationship with Health Index 2, and a further illustration that many different possible indicators of deprivation all point in the same direction in this kind of analysis, we also used multiple regression to construct a deprivation index from a wider set of variables than were used for the main Index. The first variable to enter was proportion of social class I/II households, explaining some 57 per cent of the variance, followed by car ownership and proportion of lone-pensioner households. The three together explained about 76 per cent of the variance in Health Index 2. Running the Deprivation Index in the analysis together with those indicators which do *not* form part of it, social class still entered first, followed by the Index, and the two together explained about 70 per cent of the variance. These figures are all very similar, given that the size of the multiple correlation and the order in which variables enter the equation are very unlikely to be stable with this small size of sample. The analyses confirm that deprivation is related to health status, almost however deprivation is measured, and that the Deprivation Index which we have constructed is an adequate measure. They also demonstrate, however, that despite the theoretical reasons for not adopting it discussed earlier, social class is also part of the cluster of deprivation indicators and would stand in for them if others were not available.

Health Index 1 (which used low birthweight instead of infant mortality) and the Deprivation Index were also highly correlated in the Plymouth wards – 0.86 – suggesting 74 per cent of shared variance. By comparison, the correlation of the Deprivation Index with Health Index 2 is 0.82, suggesting 67 per cent of shared variance – but the difference is probably more apparent than real, and certainly not statistically significant. Regression analysis suggested that unemployment was the prime predictor of Health Index 1, and nothing else appeared to want to contribute. However, unemployment and lack of car ownership are highly correlated in the Plymouth City wards. Again social class (proportion of class I/II households) was an equally good indicator.

Conclusions

The conclusions of this report are, firstly, there are differences in level of material deprivation between wards in the Plymouth Health Authority area. This is evident not only for the urban wards but also for rural ones, even if the factors which compose the overall Deprivation Index appear to be less predictive of rural deprivation. Secondly, there are observable differences in health experience between the wards within the PHD area, as measured by the overall Health Index employed in this study. Thirdly, there is a statistical association between wards which experience poor health status and those with high levels of deprivation. (However, this association does not hold for rural wards when analysed separately.)

Even though the South-West Regional Health Authority appears to have a better than average health status relative to the nation as a whole, this study highlights the existence of poor health status and severe material deprivation at ward level in the PHD. This pattern is corroborated by the Townsend *et al.* (1985) study of the Bristol area, in which similar instances of poverty and poor health were uncovered. Thus analysis of small geographical areas is important, since this technique highlights problem areas at local level which are often masked by the aggregation of data at regional or district levels of area analysis. Within the PHD there are specific problems of poor health in some wards, namely inner-city wards like St Peter's and Honicknowle, and rural wards are not universally healthy either (e.g. Ugborough). The distribution of material deprivation is associated with levels of ill health, and clearly these material/structural problems cannot be tackled by health service agencies in isolation.

Rural health overall does appear to be better than that of the urban areas, but since the overall Health Index in this study relies heavily on mortality statistics, perhaps the following quote from Fearn (1987) may put the problem in some perspective:

> The problem is that mortality figures may tell us that people live longer in the rural areas but they do not indicate whether rural people suffer more or less of those everyday illnesses that do not result in death and which the major part of the health services have to deal with.

Those who suffer from material deprivation, whether they live in urban or in rural areas of the PHD, do have lower life expectancies and suffer greater morbidity than the more affluent in the community. The problems which these people face have to be tackled by healthy public policy initiatives at both central and local government level.

That the association between health status and material deprivation, as measured here, seems more tenuous for rural than for urban areas suggests to us that more research is required. Car ownership, for example, was strongly correlated with health status for the PHD as a whole and for urban wards within it, but not for rural wards. This may be understood, as we have argued, but the fact remains that *no* individual indicator of material deprivation was significantly associated with rural health status – despite the fact that all the indicators are highly correlated. That deprivation and health status are *not* associated in rural areas seems unlikely. More likely is either that different measures of deprivation are needed in rural areas than in urban ones, reflecting different lifestyles and different structural factors, or that the ward is an inappropriate level of aggregation for the study of rural health status. Further research is needed to choose between these alternatives.

References

Black Report (1980). *Inequalities in Health* (eds P. Townsend and N. Davidson). Penguin, Harmondsworth.

Carstairs, V. (1981). Small area analysis and health service research. *Community Medicine*, 3, 131–139.

Craig, J. (1981). *Studies on Medical and Population Subjects*, No. 48. HMSO, London.

Cullingford, D. and Openshaw, S. (1982). Identifying areas of rural deprivation using social area analysis. *Regional Studies*, 16, 409–418.

Deacon, B. (1987). *Poverty and deprivation in the South-West: a preliminary survey from published data*. Child Poverty Action Group, London.

Fearn, R. (1987). Rural health care: a British success or a tale of unmet need? *Social Science and Medicine*, 24, 263–274.

Fox, A. J. *et al.* (1984). Approaches to studying the effect of socio-economic circumstances on geographical differences in mortality in England and Wales. *British Medical Journal*, 40, 309–314.

Hamilton-Cole, R. M. and Lang, I. (1986). *Tightening Belts*. London Food Commission, London.

Johnson, I. S. *et al.* (1987). *Health Care and Disease: a profile of Sheffield*. Sheffield Health Authority, Sheffield.

LeGrand, J. and Robinson, R. (1985). *The Economics of Social Problems*. Macmillan, London.

MacIntyre, S. (1986). The patterning of health by social position in contemporary Britain: directions for sociological research. *Social Science and Medicine*, 23, 393–415.

Marsh, G. N. and Channing, D. M. (1986). Deprivation and health in one General Practice. *British Medical Journal*, 292, 1173–1176.

Moser, K. A., Fox, A. J. and Jones, D. R. (1986). 'Unemployment and mortality in the OPCS Longtitudinal Study', in *Class and Health* (ed. R. G. Wilkinson). Tavistock, London.

OPCS (1990). *OPCS Monitor SS90/3*. Office of Population Censuses and Surveys, London.

Phillips, D. and Williams, A. (1984). *Rural Britain: a social geography*. Blackwell, Oxford.

Thunhurst, C. (1985). The analysis of small area statistics and planning for health. *Statistician*, 34, 93–106.

Townsend, P. *et al.* (1985). Inequalities in health in the city of Bristol: a preliminary review of statistical evidence. *International Journal of Health Science*, 15, 637–663.

Townsend, P. *et al.* (1986a). *Poverty and the London labour market: an interim report*. Low Pay Unit, London.

Townsend, P., Phillimore, P. and Beattie, A. (1986b). *Inequalities in health in the Northern Region: an interim report*. Northern Regional Health Authority.

Whitehead, M. (1987). *The Health Divide: inequalities in health in the 1980s*. Health Education Council, London.

Wilkinson, R. G. (1986). 'Socio-economic differences in mortality: interpreting data on their size and trends', in *Class and Health*. Tavistock, London.

Postscript

Chapter 10 gives rise to two important points about the interpretation of research results – one specific to the chapter and others of its kind, and the other more general. The specific point concerns what is known as the *ecological fallacy*, and it concerns the level of measurement being used in a study. In Chapter 10, the 'unit of account' is the Census ward, a small geographical area but one which houses a considerable number of people nonetheless. We demonstrated that some wards showed higher values of material deprivation than others (that the people in them lacked amenities, etc.), that some wards showed poorer health status (more deaths, more underweight babies, etc.), and that the two measures were correlated (the wards which had the greater deprivation also tended to have the poorer health status). The presumption must be that it was the materially deprived people who had the poorer health status. This is only a presumption, however; it could be quite different people, who just happened to have a tendency to live in the same area. Correlation does not prove causation, and it would take research at the level of people rather than wards to confirm the conclusion. The more general point is that it takes insight and imagination to look at a study and to see what it *can* show and what it *cannot*. We have to see what explanations are made possible by the design, what alternative explanations have been excluded by it, and what has been overlooked altogether. We have also to look at the setting of the study and the nature of the research subjects or informants, and to determine to what population the results can be generalized and whether they would hold true in other settings.

Another way in which imagination must be exercised, in the interpretation of research studies, is in taking account of the extent of *procedural reactivity* in the study – the extent to which the way in which it is carried out may determine the results, and the extent to which the results may be specific to that particular structured stituation. On the whole we think of experiments as the most reactive, followed by surveys, open interviewing, and then participant observation (particularly *covert* observation, where the researcher is not known to other participants as a researcher). The laboratory experiment is quite clearly a 'game', with rules, and nothing like ordinary life outside the laboratory. The structured survey is a little more like an ordinary-life event, a conversation, but it is still a very artificial conversation, and 'being interviewed' is again a game whose rules we know quite well. 'Open' interviewing is more naturalistic still, but there is still a degree of structure in the conversation, and the fact that the informants know that they are 'undergoing research' makes the situation to some extent artificial. The most naturalistic form of research is participation, where one becomes or passes as a natural participant, and this is the only style which can make serious claims to observing what goes on in real life, independently of the research context. (Its countervailing drawbacks are that it is very time-consuming, very hard and stressful work for the researcher and very dependent in its interpretation on the researcher's understanding of the situation.) The dimension of artificiality is not quite as clear-cut as we are suggesting here; a field experiment – the introduction of an experimental regime into one hospital but not another, for example – might be more naturalistic than some forms of open interviewing. Nor is it *necessarily* the case that the artificiality of the research situation makes it impossible to generalize results to 'real life'. The reader needs to consider each study on its merits, however, in the knowledge that the very structures which make the research interpretable may also diminish its generalizability.

In this last section we have looked at experiments and quasi-experimental studies whose logic mimics that of the experiment except for lack of control over the 'experimental manipulation' (being a health visitor or a social worker, in Chapter 9, or being materially deprived in Chapter 10). This is the most highly structured kind of research design, and its structure puts it in a position to der onstrate causal connections (in experiments) or at least to suggest their presence very strongly (in quasi-experimental studies). It is important to note what they *cannot* do, however. A structured study of this kind is very good for testing hypotheses, but not good at all for generating theory. In the true experiment the only factors which can emerge as explanatory variables are the experimental manipulation itself or possible a measured extraneous factor (an alternative explanation which the experiment fails to eliminate). There is no way of telling that some other kind of factor might have been more productive as an explanation, and no way of testing whether the whole explanatory framework is appropriate. An experiment about the effects of working environment on productivity can demonstrate that the environment does or does not have an effect, or that some personal or historical characteristic of the research subjects is a better explanation, but it cannot reframe the question in terms of gender or class or the prevailing economic conditions. Studies resembling Chapter 10 but with less internal structure – correlational surveys – are better for thinking round a problem and exploring it: you can collect data on a wide range of variables and look to see what correlates with what, fishing for significant patterns. The power of the study is still limited by the nature of the data collected, however; you cannot analyse what you did not collect, so the study is limited to what you already knew was important or thought might be. 'Open' techniques – open interviewing, and even more participant observation – give much more scope for the unexpected to arise as important. Even here, however, the data collected will be limited by the preconceptions of the researcher, however much he or she may try to guard against this. We must resign ourselves to the fact that theory is not generated, in the last resort, from the results of research, but from the imagination of the researcher. Empirical research is for testing theory or exploring ideas, but the ideas are not themselves a product of the research.

As we have suggested throughout this book, research is very much an act of mind, the adoption of a certain kind of imagination. A double and contrary kind of imagining is required. On the one hand, it is essential to become immersed in the topic area and the people who encapsulate it. You need to be able, to the small extent that this is possible, to think the thoughts of the participants and understand what they take for granted and why, in order to come to a realistic understanding of 'what is going on'. At the same time you need to remain marginal – to the action, to the extent that your research design permits, so that you do not disturb the natural scene more than is necessary, and to the perspectives of the participants, so that you can understand what they themselves perhaps do not understand by coming as a stranger to what they take for granted. This double marginality is a counsel of perfection and not possible of achievement, but *trying* to achieve it is the essential basis both of good research and of an informed understanding of other people's research.

This double marginality is particularly difficult to achieve when the research is concerned with our own place of work and our own professional practice. We have a 'stake' in the results, and we have to live afterwards in the place which we have analysed, both of which make for difficulties. More important, we are deeply enmeshed in the culture and expectations of the workplace and work practices; that which we are exploring and to which we are trying to remain marginal in *our own* lives and taken-for-granted ways of proceeding. To the extent that we succeed in marginalizing ourselves with respect to these, there is a terrible risk that we may *remain* marginalized – that the analysis and re-thinking involved in research will unfit us for practice at our previous level. Nonetheless, we would assert that all good practice is informed by the same kind of imagination that informs research: unexamined practice loses direction and ceases to be able to accommodate change. We therefore commend this book and the whole research enterprise to you, hoping that it does for you what it does for us – that it opens up possibilities and casts some doubt on previously undoubted certainties. Whatever else it does, we hope this book demonstrates that social research is not something arcane, the private preserve of highly trained technicians, but something we can all do for ourselves.

Author index

Subject index